INFLAMMATORY BREAST CANCER

by Verité Reily Collins

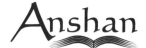

Published in the UK by:-

Anshan Ltd
11a Little Mount Sion
Tunbridge Wells
Kent. TN1 1YS

Tel: +44 (0) 1892 557767
Fax: +44 (0) 1892 530358

e-mail: info@anshan.co.uk
web site: www.anshan.co.uk

ISBN: 978 1 848290 39 6

British Library Cataloguing in Publication Data
A catalogue record for this book is available from the British Library.

Editor: Penny Worms
Cover design: Graham Rich
Cover picture: © Christine Clifford

Typeset by: Penny Worms
Printed by: Replika Press Pvt Ltd

Contents

Acknowledgements

There are so many helpful people involved in providing information for this book, and who helped me during cancer, starting with Thirza Muggleton, Jo Thompson-Hughes, Jan Lister and all the other friends who provided the most amazing and comprehensive 'care package' when I returned from hospital.

I'd also like to thank my helpful surgeon, Mr Gerald Gui, MS, FRCS, FRCS (Ed) who guided me through cancer in a calm and informative way. And I eventually ended up with a marvellous oncologist, Dr Stephen R. D. Johnston, MA, PhD, FRCP (Consultant Medical Oncologist & Reader in Breast Cancer Medicine, Director of Clinical R&D, Director of NIHR Biomedical Research Centre for Cancer, Royal Marsden NHS Foundation Trust & Institute of Cancer Research). The big title helps to explain why he is such a help to cancer patients, with all the research he undertakes and the way he translates it into understandable chunks. The informative and supportive nurses and staff on the helplines of Breast Cancer Care, Macmillan, Cancer Research UK and others. Rachel Gonzaga, Senior Health Press Officer at Cancer Research UK. Joanne from South Africa. Claire Morgan, Ann and Arthur Tait, Marina Raime of Betterdays Cancer Care Support Centre. Mirjanna, my breast nurse, who rescued me when I was in tears after being told no one had any idea why I had lost the sight in my eye. Dr Russ Hargreaves of Macmillan Centre at Chelsea and Westminster Hospital. Rosalind Stroud at Macmillan Cancer Support. Jeannie, Viv and the others who gave wonderful massages when I was undergoing treatment – you were all such a support. As were the staff at Klinic Bad Sulza in Germany and those at La Roche Posay in France. Professor Michael Baum who gave me permission to quote from his book *Breast Beating*, which he describes as a quest for an understanding of breast cancer, the meaning of life and other easy questions!

Also a big thank you to Annie Redmile, who has helped many people find their way through the benefits jungle and wrote most of Chapter 16 – Paperwork and Financial Help; Doris Lister, who helped to keep me sane; the people at Cancerkin; the happy crowd at the Paul D'Auria Cancer Support Centre in Clapham Junction –

4

always working on a shoestring and giving a wonderful service; Reverend David Brown, formerly Senior Chaplain, The Royal Marsden NHS Trust, London and Surrey; Carol Hurd, Parkside Hospital's Radiotherapy Manager; and everyone else who helped with excellent advice and information.

Reading other books on cancer, I have often been struck by how many mention US websites, even if written for British readers, and have found they go out of their way to be helpful. Writing this book, I have made 'ether friends' with many of the major US cancer hospitals and research centres (sorry, centers!). They have been incredibly informative, in particular Carolyn Grantham, Editor, dana-farber.org. Once I needed to check something my oncologist had said at a conference. Everyone at his hospital press office was 'busy', so I e-mailed Carolyn and back zipped the answer five minutes later.

Other helpful people were Nicole McMillian, MS Guidelines Coordinator National Comprehensive Cancer Network; the press office at M D Anderson; and Michael J Miller, Senior Science Writer at University of Rochester Medical Center, who went to great trouble to get me information; and Professor Edzard Ernst, MD, PhD, FRCP, FRCP (Edin.) and Dr Simon Singh and others who gave me permission to quote from their books; and finally, Christine Clifford Beckwith and Euphrosene Labon for their drawings and cartoons.

The information in this book has been gathered from many sources and while every effort has been made to ensure accuracy, please check for yourself. I can make no undertaking to its completeness or 'up-to-dateness'. However, as Carolyn Grantham kindly reassured me, basic medical information is available anywhere (more or less) but it's much harder to find those first-person tips and suggestions about how to get through the experience. This has been supplied by those whom I mention above, and others.

Verité Reily Collins

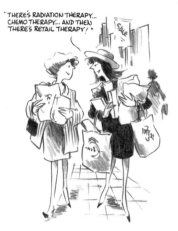

"THERE'S RADIATION THERAPY...
CHEMO THERAPY... AND THEN
THERE'S RETAIL THERAPY! "

Chapter 1

Introduction

There is one very surprising thing that comes with cancer – new friends. If you have just been diagnosed with inflammatory breast cancer (IBC), you are going to find a whole lot of new acquaintances during your cancer treatment. They will be fun to meet with, very supportive, and will even provide laughs along the way. So it's not all doom and gloom. In fact, statistics are constantly being updated and show that, every year, more and more of us are recovering and surviving.

Why read this book?

Please be aware that I am not medically qualified. If you need a book giving you the medical background to IBC, please ask your doctor or nurse. I can only give you a lay-patient's thoughts and the information I have gathered along the way.

You may have picked up this book because you are worried about an inflammation in your breast or you just have a feeling that your breast is not behaving normally. If you have looked up your symptoms on the internet, you might be wondering if you have what is known as inflammatory breast cancer. Or perhaps you have been diagnosed with this type of cancer and are feeling dazed and worried. These are normal feelings, and hopefully there will be some ideas in this book that make things easier and more positive for you. Or, you may have 'ordinary' breast cancer – and just want to know if I have any new information that might be useful for you. IBC and 'ordinary' breast cancer treatment paths are similar – just set out in a different order.

What this book offers

Here, in lay-patient's language, is:

- An explanation of the unique nature of inflammatory breast cancer
- A step-by-step idea of how your treatment will be planned, and what happens along the way
- What side effects you might have and ways to deal with them
- Hints and tips from other IBC and breast cancer survivors
- A glossary of words and terms that you might come across
- A digest of where you can get further information: reputable websites, cancer centres and cancer charities
- Contacts and more contacts

I hope it will also be something you can turn to when you want answers but when everything else seems so clinical and 'distant', or if you just need advice or reassurance.

Your doctor or nurse is the proper person with whom to discuss your symptoms. When I mention anything medical, I have included the internet source (hospitals, cancer charities, etc.), so you and your medical team can check the information. As a patient, I found that the information I was given was sometimes bewildering, written by doctors. I wanted information in simple language – not 'medic-speak'.

A few years ago, if your doctor told you that you had cancer, it was almost equivalent to a death sentence. I am not going to give you any statistics about survival rates for IBC, because the stats will have changed by the time you read this – *for the better!* Every day there are new advances in treatment, and as a specialist at the Royal Marsden Hospital said, 'miracles happen every day'.

But there is still this fear of cancer, and cancer patients are still frightened by the disease. For what it is worth, my thinking is:

- Every patient reacts differently to treatment, so there is no set standard.
- There is no template for what will happen to you during treatment.
- There is no timetable for what you have to do.
- You are you. Your body is different from any other person's, so your treatment will be different.
- You will be given drugs. No one can guarantee that you will not experience side effects with these drugs, nor what these might be, only that there *may* be side effects.
- It is the fear of the unknown that often frightens people.

However, read on. We aim to give you help, information and strategies to deal with problems.

Case stories

Throughout the book, I include stories from people who have contacted me on my website www.after-cancer.com. I started this website after a friend heard me ranting and raving about the bad service for patients in cancer hospitals. She suggested that I start a website to tell others what I had found out. The outcome was www.after-cancer.com, which was meant to 'talk' to fellow Britons, but now is the centre of a community of 131 countries (and growing). They access my jottings about what's new in the cancer field and contribute their own stories, some of which I include in this book.

The internet

Doctors and nurses are over-worked, especially in Britain, and often don't have time to talk you through the treatment. This is why so many patients turn to the internet for information. I did, and haven't looked back, so I want to encourage all those who shy away from computers or who do not have access to the internet to do the same. At first, I hated computers, until I discovered there was an enormous amount of helpful information on the web for cancer patients, easily accessible from your home. Just yesterday a friend phoned to say her grandmother, who had been diagnosed only a month before, had taken herself off to the local library for a short course on computing. She is now surfing away like mad, finding out about her treatment and loving it, even though she'd never had anything to do with 'those stupid machines' before. So, if you need to, do try to get a family member to show you how easy it is to use a computer. The staff at your local library are also very helpful. You could also take a course at an Adult Education Centre, or go to somewhere like PC World and ask someone who can speak plain English (not computer-speak) if they will give you lessons.

However, there is some bad stuff out there. If a website makes you frightened, CLOSE IT DOWN IMMEDIATELY. There are far too many 'baddies' out there, preying on our fears, trying to get you to buy a product or sign up to their treatment regime. If you are worried, phone one of the cancer charity helplines (see chapter 18). They will reassure you and give you accurate information.

And where I mention websites, I have tried to put in phone numbers, just in case you don't believe me when I say how much fun computers can be!

Getting help

Almost every cancer has special drugs, and each has side effects. Everyone reacts differently to these drugs, and patients have a fear of the unknown. But knowing where to find sensible and helpful information about problems can take away fears. So in this book, I aim to set out the main points on your treatment path, and *if* you get side effects, inform you of the medically-approved methods of treating them.

Patients are often far too timid to ask for help when dealing with side effects, such as hot flushes or peeling skin. Over-worked doctors may simply say, 'Do you want to come off the drug?' Instead, they should say, 'I am sending you to Dr X who knows all about this', as happens in countries with better post-cancer survival rates. If you are just starting out on your treatment path, you are going to have to be ASSERTIVE – not argumentative, as you want the medics on your side, but show them that IBC hasn't affected your brain and you want to be referred to someone who can help. Time and time again doctors tell me that demanding patients have the better survival rates!

If you come across doctors who don't listen to you, imagine what doctors and nurses who have been diagnosed with breast cancer say about their fellow medics! When Reverend David Brown was Senior Chaplain at the Royal

Marsden Hospital, he said doctors were constantly coming to him for advice because they didn't know how to talk to patients. So make it easy for them. Tell them clearly and slowly that you don't understand what they are saying, and could they tell you again please. One patient was so horrified at the way her doctor handled her diagnosis that she went back and suggested that he needed training in how to deliver the news – and she was the person to do it. She ended up marrying him and says he's a much better doctor now!

Information sources

I quote many sources, such as hospitals, cancer centres and cancer charities. This is not laziness! It is so you can see all the positive work that is being done throughout the world to help us and improve outcomes. Naming the source is not only polite, but it gives you a contact to find out more.

Alternative treatments

If you are interested in alternative treatments, this book is not for you. Sadly, even though there are many books about alternative treatments, very often those people who follow them don't survive. What they decide to take probably hasn't been clinically proven – it is just someone's idea or theory. If everything else fails, there is nothing to stop you from trying an alternative or unusual treatment, but I don't recommend anything in this book. The reason why doctors advocate the conventional chemotherapy, surgery, radiotherapy and hormonal drugs pathway is because this is proven to work for the vast majority of people.

So in this book I have mentioned different products and therapies for the following reasons:

- There have been clinical trials to prove the product works
- The product is approved by reputable cancer treatment centres
- It is a therapy that is recommended by a cancer charity or cancer centre, with proof that it works
- It has been approved by the FDA (food and drug agency) of the country.

My 'hero' products

Some nurses will be horrified by the number of products I mention. I make no apology for this. It seems okay for the medical profession to accept funding from drug companies to carry out clinical trials (they wouldn't be able to afford to run them otherwise). And it seems okay for doctors to put us on the drugs that come through these trials, but when it comes to asking for help in dealing with the resulting side effects, the medical professionals becomes all pious, and say, 'I couldn't possibly recommend anything commercial.' Well, I don't share these ethics and I *can* mention commercial products that have helped me and my friends. If this 'advertising' offends – just turn the page! However, I don't mention any of the thousands of 'miracle pills', crystal therapies and other treatments out there. The only PR puffs I pay any attention to are those that tell me that chocolate might be good for my health. Now, there's my weakness!

Good luck with your treatment, and if needed, BE ASSERTIVE!

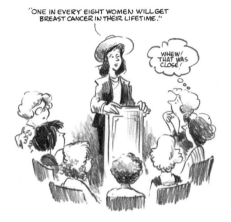

Chapter 2

What is inflammatory breast cancer?

Inflammatory breast cancer (IBC) is an advanced and accelerated form of breast cancer, not usually detected by mammograms or ultrasounds. It is a very unusual form of breast cancer, with only a small percentage of women presenting with this – and a minute amount of men. Yes, men can get breast cancer too – but as Cancer Research UK says, it is very rare. The American Cancer Society says IBC tends to occur in younger women, and African-American women appear to be at higher risk of IBC than white women.

You don't have to have a lump to have cancer. Because of the way IBC grows and spreads, a distinct lump may not be noticeable during a clinical breast exam, breast self-exam, or even on a mammogram. However, signs of IBC can be seen on the surface of the skin. Skin thickening often does show up on a mammogram and can be seen during a breast exam. Symptoms of IBC can develop very quickly, so women should pay attention to how the skin on their breasts looks, and tell their doctors *immediately* about any changes in skin texture or breast appearance. Turn over for a list of possible symptoms.

It is very important to distinguish inflammatory breast cancer from other types of breast cancer, because there are major differences in its symptoms, prognosis, and treatment. IBC requires immediate aggressive treatment. So if you feel uneasy about your body, or are not sure you have been given a correct diagnosis, **ask immediately for a second opinion.** Don't think you are being stupid or awkward by asking for this – many of us owe our lives to the fact that we queried a diagnosis. We KNOW our bodies, so if we think we have something, chances are we are right. Singer Kylie Minogue admits she was misdiagnosed at first. She went back and insisted on more tests, and it was discovered that she did have breast cancer. In its early stages, IBC can be diagnosed as mastitis; a breast infection, for which you are prescribed antibiotics. If there is no improvement after you have taken the antibiotics for a week, ask immediately for a biopsy or to be referred on.

Don't believe old wives' tales that you can't have breast cancer whilst pregnant or feeding. Many have their first symptoms during this time, and IBC on average presents earlier than 'ordinary' breast cancer – the average age at diagnosis for IBC is six years earlier.

Symptoms

Inflammatory breast cancer is so named because the top or overlying layer of breast skin often has a red, inflamed appearance. It looks similar to the symptoms you get with breast infections. The inflammation takes place because IBC spreads along and blocks the lymph vessels in the skin of the breast, leading to an obstruction in the lymph flow. Lymph vessels are responsible for removing fluid and other waste products from the body's tissues to help prevent infections.

According to Breast Cancer Care (BCC):

'In patients with IBC, the reddened appearance is caused by breast cancer cells blocking tiny channels in the breast tissue called lymph channels. The lymph channels are part of the lymphatic system involved in the body's defence against infection.'

MD Anderson, one of the top cancer hospitals in the world, has established a clinic specially to treat IBC. They say many women don't get proper treatment until the disease is well-advanced, and therefore harder to treat.

Most authorities agree the most common symptoms are one or perhaps a combination of these:

- warmth or heat in the breast
- redness, red or pink skin
- swelling
- soreness
- rash (from a small patch to across the entire breast)
- ridges in the skin
- the breast may appear pitted
- the breast may look like the skin of an orange (often called by the French term *peau d'orange*)
- a lump or lumps
- pain in the breast or nipple
- itchiness in the breast
- nipple discharge
- the nipple may be inverted (turned invward)
- one breast larger than the other
- swollen lymph nodes under the armpit or on the neck

Symptoms can appear over a very short space of time, so if you even think you might have IBC, or have any of these symptoms, it is vital to see your doctor immediately. If your doctor prescribes antibiotics, **all the authorities say that, if a reaction to the antibiotics is not obvious after a week, then a biopsy should be undertaken or a medical appointment with a breast authority is warranted.** In spite of its name, inflammatory breast cancer does not lead to inflammation in the same way an infection does. So, to repeat, if you still have:

- rapid alteration in the appearance of one breast, in the course of days or weeks
- thickness, heaviness or noticeable swelling of one breast
- discoloration, giving the breast a red, purple, pink or black-and-blue appearance

- atypical warmness in the affected breast
- dimpling or ridges on the skin of the affected breast, akin to orange peel
- itching
- tenderness, pain or aching
- enlarged lymph nodes under the arm
- a flattened or inward-turning nipple
- alteration in the colour of the skin around the nipple

Go back to your doctor and ask for a second opinion!

IBC happens to people all over the world. Joanne from South Africa says:

'I was diagnosed aged 42. My symptom was a red and swollen left boob. It was very tender to touch, like mastitis, which is what I thought it was. One doctor actually asked me if I had been bitten by an insect! I went to my gynaecologist for his opinion. He referred me to a surgeon who did a biopsy ... It was IBC.'

Valerie says:

'I woke up one morning and just knew something was wrong. Luckily I have a doctor who says, "I listen to my women patients – they know their own bodies." So when I went to see him that evening he didn't laugh at me, but instead sent me off for tests. He said he couldn't find anything, but believed me when I said I knew something didn't feel right. And something was wrong, so luckily he listened to me.'

It can be difficult to diagnose IBC. The symptoms can be similar to a breast infection, but breast infections typically arise during breast-feeding. With an infection, you'll probably also have a fever, which is atypical of IBC. Luckily, as our medical knowledge improves, more and more doctors and nurses are becoming familiar with this uncommon type of cancer.

So go back to your doctor and demand an investigation for IBC if you have any slight suspicion that you might have it. According to so many who have had it, there are still dinosaurs around who deny there is such a thing. You need to be assertive and quietly remind them that it is your right to have a second opinion. After all, if you are proven to have made a fuss over nothing, so what? It's your life – look after yourself!

Facts about IBC

IBC is an unusual cancer, and only 1–2 per cent (one or two patients in one hundred) of breast cancers are IBC. In the USA, IBC accounts for 1–5 per cent of all breast cancer cases, and in North Africa possibly around 7 per cent.

As it is rare, it can go undiagnosed by doctors for a long time. However, you need to be aware that this form of cancer can be aggressive, so it needs to be attended to quickly. **Although rare, it is treatable**, and there is on-going research to find out more about it and its treatment.

- It tends to be diagnosed in younger women, compared to non-IBC breast cancer.
- It occurs more frequently and at a younger age in African-Americans than in Whites.
- Like other types of breast cancer, IBC can occur in men, but usually at an older age than in women.

Although it is a more serious form of breast cancer, Breast Cancer Care say *'treatment continues to improve, which means that the outcome may be more positive now than in the past'.*

Breast cancer has been around for a long time. One of the earliest medical documents is known as the Edwin Smith Papyrus. Edwin Smith was an Egyptologist who bought the manuscript in Egypt in 1862. Although he understood its importance of it, he never published the papyrus and it was all but forgotten. It wasn't until the 20th century that this document was rediscovered. Dating back to 1600 BC, it is our first known medical writing and it is important to the history of breast cancer because it describes in writing the earliest known cases of the disease – one of which was a man. An ancient Egyptian doctor wrote, *'There is no treatment.'* We have come a long way since then, and every day provides a new treatment or a step along the way to a cure.

North Africa

If you or your family come from Tunisia, Egypt and any nearby North African country, recent research by bodies such as the World Health Organization has identified that this type of breast cancer may be seen more often in women from this region.

A recent report, *Inflammatory Breast Cancer in Tunisia: Reassessment of Incidence and Clinicopathological Features* by Hamouda Boussen and others, says:

> Inflammatory breast cancer is a clinical diagnosis characterized by a peculiar geographic distribution in incidence, being particularly common in Tunisia and the region of North Africa. The peculiar aspects of the disease in this region may provide some insights on the biological characteristics of the disease. We updated and revised the data from our single-institution experience using the more stringent diagnostic criteria of the International Union Against Cancer (UICC) based on the tumour-node-metastasis (TNM) classification.

> Interestingly, using a more uniform classification criteria, the incidence of IBC was 5% to 7% compared to previous historical reports of up to 50% of newly diagnosed cases of breast cancer in Tunisia.

> Our study reflects the difficulty in diagnosing true IBC and differentiating it from LABC or neglected breast cancer. Despite a decrease in the incidence of IBC in Tunisia after reassessment to around 7%, it remains higher than the 1% to 2% reported in western countries.

> *Semin Oncol 35:17-24 © 2008 Elsevier Inc. All rights reserved.*

What tests may be used to identify IBC?

Probably one or more of the following:

- Preliminary manual examination of the breast by a doctor
- Mammogram
- Breast ultrasound (sonography or ultrasonography)

- MUGA scan (Multiple Gated Acquisition Scan) to check the heart
- Chest X-ray to check the lungs, heart and chest wall
- Bone scan (radionuclide scan) to check the bones
- CAT scan, PET scan, and MRI to check soft tissue, bones and blood vessels

Then you may be given one or more of the following to take sample breast tissue. Skin biopsies are helpful in some cases. The type of procedure depends on where the affected area is, what it looks like, and who finds it:

- fine-needle aspiration biopsy (FNA)
- core needle biopsy
- vacuum-assisted biopsy
- large core biopsy
- punch biopsy
- surface biopsy
- open surgical biopsy (excisional and incisional).

Having a biopsy

Some women find breast biopsies painful, but as Valerie says:

> *'I think that the "pain" could come from the worry. I was given an injection to numb my breast, and then the doctor took various samples – no pain at all.'*

Paget's Disease

The symptoms for Paget's Disease can sometimes cause confusion. If this develops into cancer – although the disease is dissimilar – treatment often follows the same path. See more in the glossary, on page 159, or go to the Breast Cancer Care website www.breastcancercare.org.uk/upload/pdf/pagets.

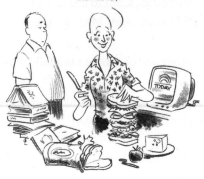

Chapter 3
Diagnosis

After Valerie had her biopsy, she returned to the hospital for the results:

> *'You've got to laugh. I knew immediately that I had cancer when I arrived at the hospital. As soon as I gave my name, the receptionist actually looked up from her screen, and instead of barking "wait over there", she cracked a smile and said, "Nurse Jane will look after you." Total giveaway. So Nurse Jane, holding her box of tissues, took me into the doctor's room. By this time my mind was in overdrive, so the doctor was faced with a patient who didn't want any tissues, but did want to know, "When are you going to operate?"'*

One poor friend burst into tears. She had been shown into a room with a surgeon, other team members, and someone who was introduced as 'our Macmillan nurse'. As soon as she heard those words, she was convinced this meant she was going to die – as far as she knew, Macmillan nurses only looked after the terminally ill. Today, however, Macmillan nurses are around in many hospitals, supporting the breast care team, and carrying out different roles.

After receiving her diagnosis, Valerie said:

'This was where me and the NHS system parted company. The doctor told me, "You will see a doctor within two weeks." (Translation: "This will get us off the hook in meeting our Government targets and we can wait weeks before you see a surgeon to get a date for an op.") No thanks.'

Luckily waiting times have improved dramatically, and it is unlikely that you will have to wait more than a few days. However, if the wait is too long and you are worried sick, and if you don't have private insurance, go back to your GP, tell him or her your fears, and ask for a fast-track appointment. If they are reluctant to do this, you can phone the secretary of the doctor with whom you have your appointment and ask if there is a cancellation. If there isn't, ask if you can call again. If you are nice, they are often very helpful.

Claire's Story is from a website:

'I was diagnosed with inflammatory breast cancer at the age of 34, about six weeks after I first noticed something might be wrong. In early January I noticed my left breast was red and hot to the touch. The nipple was also inverted, but as this was around the time of my period I ignored it. In my defence of this action I would say I had an awful lot going on in my family life. At the beginning of February, I thought I should get it checked out, but wasn't particularly concerned, thinking it was just an infection. I saw my GP on the Friday evening. On seeing my breast, he immediately knew it was serious. I was referred to the breast clinic at St George's Hospital and was seen the following Wednesday. All the tests were completed that day and by the end of the day I had a firm diagnosis of breast cancer. Further tests on the biopsy were needed to indicate what kind. I returned to the clinic the following Wednesday and was told the cancer was inflammatory breast cancer, and the advised treatment was chemotherapy, followed by a mastectomy and finally radiotherapy. I was to start chemo the following week, so all-in-all, from the initial visit to the GP to starting

chemotherapy was three weeks.

With hindsight I can now see that in those first couple of months I was in shock. Everything happened so quickly, but I thought this was normal. Everyone said how well I was coping, but in truth I was on auto-pilot, relying on the medical team to tell me what to do.

It was only half way through my six cycles of chemo, that I found out that inflammatory breast cancer was indeed very bad news (this was in 2001), but by then my treatment was progressing well, so worrying about it seemed pointless. I must say I'm glad I wasn't in full possession of all the facts at the start because some of those facts made pretty grim reading.'

Claire's comment about being on 'auto-pilot' describes exactly how most patients feel. Doctors should take note of this and, instead of giving us long talks about the course of action, should leave this until later when we have got over the shock and can take in what they are saying. If you find yourself on auto-pilot, try asking the doctor for an appointment in a few weeks when you can ask the questions. Treating cancer takes a long time, so there is space to give yourself some time to get back into the real world.

And what Claire says about treatment in 2001 is no longer relevant. IBC has been the subject of many studies, more is known about it, and the treatment is progressing all the time.

Your first visit

Once your diagnosis has been confirmed, you will start on the treatment path. During this time it is quite normal to be in a total daze. We have all heard horror stories of cancer but don't know what is going to happen. We are fearful for the future. Your specialist is going to hopefully reassure you. You will meet nurses who are full of sensible information, and this is when friends start to offer help. Don't turn them down. You may feel you don't want to talk to anyone. Tell them you are just not able to think at the moment, but can they contact you in a week when you have heard about your treatment plan. You really do want them to do this, as supportive friends can be incredibly useful.

Notebook

In the time leading up to your first visit to see your oncologist (the doctor or surgeon who is going to look after you), it is natural for 'What if?' thoughts to fill your head. You will suddenly think of something that is important to you, or that you need an explanation for – so it helps to invest in a small notebook to carry with you at all times. Jot down questions as they come into your head. Then, while you are waiting to see the specialist, underline those that are of particular concern. If they are there, in black and white, you won't forget to ask.

We are all fearful for the future, but writing down things that worry you can often transfer your worries into a book – and it helps.

Taking a friend

When you have your appointment to tell you what you've got and how it is to be treated, you may be asked to bring a friend. There are pros and cons:

PROS

- You will be in a state of shock, so it is helpful to have someone with you to take you home.
- The theory is that two heads remember the diagnosis better than one (but see below).
- Your friend can take notes and discuss these with you afterwards.

CONS

- You may feel you can't discuss intimate matters in front of a friend, however close they are.
- You want to be in control during your treatment, and may find it difficult to ask questions in front of someone else.
- The theory is that you and your friend can discuss the diagnosis afterwards, but chances are that if you haven't understood something, your friend won't have either, and you are left putting your heads together to try to guess what the specialist meant.

Valerie says:

'I was very unpopular. Told to bring a friend, when I arrived on my own

the nurse . . . seemed put out that I had come alone. But I wanted to take time to discuss **me** *with the specialist. I didn't want to have to think that this was boring for a friend, or if we were kept waiting, would this make her late? And I might be embarrassed to discuss medical matters, even in front of my best friend. I wanted to go over and over the diagnosis with the specialist, repeating and asking questions, so at the end of the appointment I came out understanding totally what was going to happen. Also, I got the impression that with two people in front of a specialist, he could blind them with science and they would both escape thinking "the other one will understand".'*

So think carefully – friends are very important, but for that first appointment a partner who understands you and the way you think is probably the best person to have there. Failing that, decide if you really want anyone with you, or if you want to explore all the options until you understand them.

Sometimes the medical profession needs help in handling us. Professor Michael Baum is a very eminent breast surgeon, and commented recently about *"young doctors who know all about molecular biology on the one hand or managing a fund-holding practice on the other, but little about the feelings of the patient in the middle!"* Anyone can die from cancer, but today, even if you have cancer, you are far more likely to die from an age-related condition – not the cancer. If you have confidence in your specialist, and if they have a good reputation among their medical peers, you can rest assured that they have been there, seen it and know what works. They will probably have participated in clinical trials (more about these later), so they have seen at first-hand what is effective, and had this confirmed with rigorous, medically-supervised trials. Some drugs that have come through these trials could almost be classed as miracle drugs. You only have to compare the survival charts of 20 to 30 years ago (when cancer was a taboo word, as it was almost certainly a killer disease) with post-cancer survival rates today.

After diagnosis

More than likely you will be sent a copy of a follow-up letter the specialist will send to your doctor. This letter will be full of the medical terms for what is wrong with you. There is a glossary at the end of the book (page 147) to help you decipher letters such as these, and if you want, you can go on the internet to find out more.

In the past, there was a lot of scepticism about information on the internet. Today, provided you are sensible, this information can be of tremendous benefit. Websites of Macmillan, Cancer Research UK, or the great American cancer hospitals, such as Dana Farber, MD Anderson, Sloane-Kettering (web addresses in chapter 18) have sections for medics and for patients. They know that patients want informed advice, so it will be there, written in a language you can understand!

If you find a website is trying to sell you something (unless you have gone on to the site to actually buy a product), click on to the next one.

Also, avoid the blogs that give you a gloomy picture. Yes, cancer can be a bugger (if you'll pardon the expression), but there is lots of help out there, so look for that. Try to avoid the 'I cured my cancer by ...' blogs that advocate everything from grapes to crystals. Sadly, many of the people who write these books claiming to have been cured are no more. If eating goji berries, drinking aloe vera juice or sitting under a crystal tent really cured cancer, hospitals would be stocking these and offering them to patients. Until they do, treat these claims with extreme caution.

Guilty? Me?

Some patients have horrid guilt feelings, convincing themselves that their cancer is their fault. **This is absolute nonsense.** Take the worst scenario – although smoking is one of the known causes of cancer, it doesn't follow that because you smoke you will get cancer. Some people who get lung cancer have never smoked in their lives.

So how do you get cancer?

Cancer Research UK says:

> 'Often, chance plays a big part. Some people are more prone to developing a cancer because of the genes they inherited at birth.

This is hardly something you, or anyone else, has any control over. But most cancers are not due to an inherited gene. Cancers start because of a mistake in copying DNA when normal cells are dividing and growing. Several of these mistakes have to happen before a cell becomes cancerous. Although some of our unhealthy behaviour can increase the risk of these mistakes, they can also just happen by chance. Cancer being "just one of those things" is something that some people really struggle with. It doesn't help to answer those "why me" questions that most people have."

As happened with me, my mother and my grandmother had breast cancer, my father had prostate cancer, and various uncles and aunts had cancer, too. But my surgeon said my type of breast cancer had NOT been inherited from anyone.

So, since chance plays its part, and doctors rarely know exactly what has caused a cancer, there's no reason to blame yourself or others. If you feel this way, phone one of the cancer charity helplines (see chapter 18) – and listen to their wise advice.

What happens next?

Once you have had your first appointment confirming IBC, treatment usually starts straight way. IBC can grow more quickly than other types of cancer, so doctors want to do what they can to prevent cells spreading to other parts of the body.

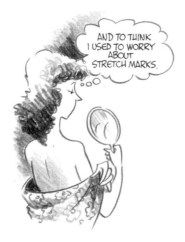

Chapter 4

Chemotherapy

For the next few weeks or months you will be going down a well-researched path, with one step following another. After diagnosis you will be referred to an oncology surgeon (the person who will operate on you). The surgeon will work in tandem with the oncologist (the person who supervises the drug treatments you will receive). They will supervise your treatment, and map out what is going to happen to you. Then, with any luck, you will be introduced to your oncology nurse – sometimes a breast care or Macmillan nurse. These people are worth their weight in gold. They literally know it all and help you to make sense of what is happening.

Every patient is different. Even if you and a friend were diagnosed with the same cancer at the same time, it doesn't follow that you would both have the same treatment at the same time – or even at different times. There are lots of factors to take into consideration. Your oncologist will be weighing these up. You will eventually be told what is going to happen, but things may change, depending how you react to drugs. Just expect the unexpected. You have had the worst news – 'You've got cancer' – so now you can cope with anything.

Multi-disciplinary teams (MDT)

There will be **multi-disciplinary team** (MDT) meetings about you. Funnily enough, you are the most important component but you will never be part of these meetings. This is just how it is, and you will probably be too dazed anyway to ask sensible questions. Save them for later, when you do know what you are talking about and can challenge the medics if need be. But don't worry. They know what they are doing. They've seen it all before, so have confidence in your team – you are in very good hands. If you *don't* have confidence in the team, now is the time to say so. Don't think that the conveyor belt has started and you can't stop it. You can. It's your life and your body. If you need to ask questions, do so. And, hopefully, someone will realize they have been taking you for granted, and take time to explain what is going on. If no one pays you any attention, a good old-fashioned tantrum might be called for – just once – to show your team that you are alive, have feelings and YOU WANT TO KNOW. Then you can jump back on the conveyor belt, feeling that you are more in control. You'll also know who you can ask if something isn't clear, and you will probably find that the team will actually start talking to you and explaining things. They will be frightened of you having another tantrum!

Professor Aidan Halligan, ex-Director of Clinical Governance at the NHS, speaks plain English, not medical speak. At a recent Macmillan conference, he said, *'Doctors must learn to communicate,'* and illustrated this by telling the story of Bill, who had just had an angiogram (an X-ray of his heart): *'That evening his consultant came into the ward, and pointed to patients saying, "You are a triple. You're a triple." Coming to Bill, he said, "You're a single." Poor Bill was mortified – he was only a "single", whatever that meant.'* For those of us who don't understand 'medic speak', the fewer bypasses a patient has to have the better. So Bill's diagnosis was more favourable – but no one told him that!

Treating inflammatory breast cancer

Treatment is usually slightly different for IBC than ordinary breast cancer. Usually the treatment path is:

- chemotherapy

- surgery
- radiotherapy
- hormone therapy

The Inflammatory Breast Cancer Research Council says:

'While the most common order of the treatment protocol is chemotherapy, surgery, more chemotherapy, and radiation, treatment options vary from doctor to doctor, from institution to institution, and can be based on geography, your individual medical history, and on the stage or progression of your cancer at the time of diagnosis.'

Everyone reacts differently, and your oncologist might decide to change the treatment path, so again expect the unexpected. You have the right to call a halt and ask what is happening any time you feel frightened, worried or don't understand.

Fear

I often think that with cancer it is probably the fear of the unknown that gives everyone such a dread of the disease. When you have a broken leg or a heart operation, treatment follows a well-defined path. But with cancer, it is different for everyone. However, if you need cheering up, remember that cancer survival rates, almost without fail, have consistently risen; things get better all the time.

Chemotherapy

Chemotherapy, or chemo for short, is generally the first treatment you will have. If you want to show off with long words, this is neoadjuvant chemotherapy. Adjuvant means 'giving additional support'. Neoadjuvant therapy is treatment given as a first step to shrink a tumour before the main treatment, which is usually surgery. Examples of neoadjuvant therapy include chemotherapy, radiation therapy, and hormone therapy. Chemotherapy actually means the use of chemical agents to treat or control diseases such as cancer. People dread this treatment, and in the old days there were some horrendous stories. Today, treatments are less harsh, and if one chemo drug doesn't agree with you, you may be able to change to a different cocktail of drugs.

How it works

Your oncologist will work with the pharmacist and nurses to ensure the best and most suitable drug or drugs are administered. That is why you often have to wait around during treatment, as every patient has to have different drugs, with time taken to check and dispense for each patient, and your dose might change according to how you are reacting.

The chemo drug travels through the body, attacking cells that are dividing quickly. Normal cells divide at a rate that is tightly controlled; however, in cancer cells this process goes wrong and results in uncontrolled production of new cells and the formation of a tumour or blood cancer.

Chemo is actually shorthand for 'cytotoxic chemotherapy' – the cytotoxics being the main group of drugs used against cancer. Cytotoxic means 'cell poison', and this describes what they do. So when cancer cells come to reproduce they are blocked from doing so and die off. Serves 'em right!

The downside is that currently most chemo drugs can't tell the difference between good and bad cells, so they zap nice cells as well as bad. Hence the nasty side effects. The good news is that good cells usually recover from effects of chemo more quickly than cancer cells. This is why chemo is often given in short courses, with intervals in between, to allow normal cells to recover without lasting injury.

If you are interested, BUPA (the private medical health insurance company) has a very informative site. They say most chemotherapy affects the DNA in cancer cells:

> 'DNA is the chemical that stores the genetic information in a cell. It controls what a cell does, including how it divides. By affecting the DNA, most chemo drugs interfere with the division of cancer cells and may cause the cancer to die back completely.'

Chemo treatment

When you start chemo treatment, you can feel you are on a conveyor belt.

Doctors, nurses, technicians and other unidentified people will introduce themselves to you, examine you, ask questions, make notes, then drift off again. You may never see them again, but the questions they ask you will go towards determining what treatment options you will be given.

Generally, you will get chemo treatment as an outpatient. Sometimes you drink the drug, but often you sit in a comfortable chair and a nurse will insert a hollow needle into a vein. This is attached to a line attached to a plastic bag that drips the chemo drugs into your veins. It sounds horrendous, but most nurses are experts at inserting the needles almost painlessly – promise! Today needles are thinner, nurses are kinder, and painkillers are used more. If you don't like what is happening when they come along and stick things in you, TELL THEM. There are lots of numbing treatments they can give you, so do ask.

Make a friend of your breast care or oncology nurse. Your nurse is the person who should give you support, help you to manage side effects, or suggest to your MDT (see page 28) that you need a different drug. If you are in a hospital without such a nurse, and feel you have no one to whom you can ask day-to-day questions, march into the Administrative Offices and demand to know why. One bad side of private treatment is some hospitals skimp on these services; it was several weeks after my operation that I discovered the Cromwell Hospital should have introduced me to 'my' nurse. When I transferred to the Royal Marsden, I had to go through the process again, and there were vague 'Oh! You are private' murmurs. Finally, a long time later, I was 'given' a nurse to contact. It took time, and I felt that I had been foisted on her and had added to her workload.

Pain

Everyone dreads this, but often the anticipation is worse than the reality. Many people don't experience any pain at all, but if it comes, this can be after treatment – sometimes a day or two later. Ask your doctor and nurse beforehand about what you can do for pain relief. Most are kind and caring, and don't want you to suffer any pain at all; but just in case yours happens to be one of the old-fashioned ones, get your action plan sorted out first.

Today, there are many ways of controlling pain. To find what is best for you:

- Talk to your doctor about the type of medication that is best for your condition – some painkillers might react with drugs you already take.
- You and your doctor should discuss other methods of controlling pain, including exercises, acupuncture, massage and more.
- Don't suffer in silence. How can anyone help if you don't tell them you are in pain?
- If not adequately managed, pain may have a tremendous effect on your quality of life.
- Don't be British about it – none of this stiff upper lip. Fighting off pain is counter-productive and uses energy and resources that should be aimed at getting you better.
- Always notify your doctor if you have pain or if your existing pain increases. Your doctor can help you find the medication or combination of medications, and the correct dosage, to control your pain. Always take your pain medication as prescribed.

Treating pain with drugs

Doctors rate pain on a scale of 1 to 10, with 1 being no pain and 10 being the worst pain. Based on this scale, the World Health Organization has outlined guidelines that your doctor may follow:

- **Mild-to-moderate pain (1-3):** your doctor may recommend over-the-counter medications.
- **Moderate-to-severe pain (4-6):** your doctor may prescribe an opioid, also known as narcotics. Opioids are similar to natural substances produced by the body to control pain, called endorphins. These are the strongest pain relievers available.
- **Severe pain (7-10):** your doctor may prescribe a stronger opioid.

Your doctor may also recommend adding a non-opioid analgesic or a supporting drug as needed. This can be given in various ways:

- Pill or liquid (oral)
- Ointment or patch (topical)
- Suppository (rectal)

- Injection into your vein (IV, or intravenous)

If your doctor gives you pain medication with instructions to 'take as needed' take it before the pain becomes severe. Medication takes time to work. Wait too long, and it may not kick in quickly enough to be effective.

Extended-release medicines

If your pain relief does not last long enough, ask your doctor about extended-release medicines, which can control pain for a longer period of time. Morphine and oxycodone are made in extended-release forms. Also, a skin patch that releases the opioid fentanyl can be used.

Concerns

Your doctors and nurses will be keeping a careful monitoring eye on you, to ensure you don't become addicted. In some cases it may be possible to map out when your up and down days will be during treatment. Go to www.breastcancer.org/treatment/chemotherapy/planning_for.jsp for more information.

Clinical trials

You may be invited to take part in trials of a new drug. These, and their possible outcome, need to be discussed carefully and thoroughly with your doctor. Clinical trials are research studies in which people agree to try new therapies (under careful supervision) in order to help doctors identify the best treatments with the fewest side effects. These studies help to improve the overall standard of care. Today, fewer than 5 per cent of breast cancer patients receive treatment for their disease in a clinical trial. Why? One reason is that information about current trials and how to enrol in one are often not understood.

For more information, the Breastcancer.org website, www.breastcancer.org, has the following details:

- What clinical trials are
- Why clinical trials are important
- How clinical trials are conducted
- Who can participate in a clinical trial

- How long do clinical trials last
- Who conducts clinical trials and who pays for them
- The different stages (phases) of clinical trials
- Benefits and risks of participating in a clinical trial
- What you should know before deciding to be part of a clinical trial
- How to find clinical trials
- Definition of terms used to talk about clinical trials

And Cancer Research UK has an excellent list of current clinical trials on www.cancerhelp.org.uk/trials.

Dr Andrew Lawson, consultant at the Royal Berkshire Hospital, wrote an article in the *Sunday Times* about what he did after he was told he had a 'supposedly incurable cancer'. He described how he went to the USA to take part in clinical trials, *'but the chances are that, if you were a cancer patient, your NHS doctor would not even have told you such a trial existed.'* The trials are completely funded by the US Government and all he had to do was pay for travel and board. He went on to say, *'Why shouldn't patients in the NHS be able to try such innovative trials in the US – or elsewhere . . . it is not so much a question of cost as a willingness to embrace new ideas.'*

However, you should think carefully before deciding to enter clinical trials. Generally, they are of tremendous benefit to patients and you are less likely to suffer side effects because the drug companies often pay for nurses to come to your home and help alleviate them. However, there have been problems with drugs trials in the past. TeGenero was an anti-inflammatory drug trialled in Britain in 1996. Six participants developed the most horrendous symptoms and ended up in intensive care. Animal trials had been successful, so this extreme and sudden reaction in humans was completely unexpected.

So, before you decide to join any clinical trial, do careful research and ask questions.

Fertility

If you are fertile before treatment begins and you want to preserve your options to have children, don't start treatment without first asking how this will affect your future plans. **Don't wait until you have finished treatment to find that your ability to conceive is gone.** You do have choices, but you must discuss ways of trying to preserve your fertility with your doctor. The major cancer charities have information on their websites, and new discoveries and ways of treating are being tried constantly.

Treatment at home

In certain circumstances you might be able to arrange treatment at home. A company called Healthcare at Home can arrange this.

Cheryl Vidall, their Clinical Risk and Practice Development Manager, says:

'Nursing a patient with inflammatory breast cancer can be challenging for the family and the healthcare professionals. There is very little time between diagnosis and chemotherapy commencing (usually a few days). The care, knowledge and understanding from nurses providing this service needs to be of the highest standard. Healthcare at Home nurses have many years' experience of managing inflammatory breast cancer and can respond to the changing needs of all involved in the care pathway. Home care has been readily available for those who have private medical insurance but is becoming more widely available on the NHS. If patients know to ask for it, their consultant may be able to access the local team for care at home, if this would be appropriate.

As a nurse working for Healthcare at Home, I find that the treatment is well tolerated at home, with one-to-one personalized care delivered. Nurses always stay for the whole infusion and are experienced in chemotherapy delivery in the home. The local nursing team offers 24-hour on-call support for patients receiving chemotherapy, providing reassurance 365 days of the year.

Healthcare at Home strives to continually improve on the patient experience. Our satisfaction surveys repeatedly give us valuable comments from patients, some of which are found below.

- *"More convenient than having to travel to hospital."*
- *"Costs me less time and money than travelling to hospital."*
- *"Comfort, reassurance, reduced stress of treatment in home*

environment."
- *"Easier to have family around if I want them there."*
- *"Less reliant on others for transport, childcare, etc."*
- *"One-to-one undivided attention of an experienced nurse throughout the treatment."*
- *"Same nurse for most visits so we build up a relationship."*

In the last five years we have treated over 10,000 cancer patients.

For more information contact info@hahGroup.

Side effects

Every drug affects people in different ways. Sometimes you will receive just one drug; other cancers are treated with a cocktail of drugs. If you can't tolerate one drug, there is generally another that can be administered. Some patients are lucky, and have few or even no side effects. I hope you are one of these lucky ones. If you are not, ask for help. So often cancer patients just curl up into their own world, and don't give others a chance to help. See Chapters 9 (page 66) and 18 (page 135) for ideas that might help with handling some side effects.

Here are the most common side effects you may experience during chemotherapy:

- tiredness
- nausea
- loss of hair
- weight gain
- changes in appetite and taste
- diarrhoea or constipation
- skin or nail problems

Recent research has highlighted that side effects from the drugs are often under-reported. Now is the time to realize that if you have side effects, you MUST make these known to your team. In many cases there is something that can be done – or even a drug can be changed to another that may not have that effect on you. I am repeating this mantra over and over again because medical staff are so busy that unless you make your point loudly and clearly, your concerns could be overlooked.

Losing Hair

Probably what worries most people is losing their hair. Yet those who have lost hair seem surprisingly relaxed about it, especially as it usually grows back quickly. If it happens to you, the NHS or charities will usually provide a wig, and if these make you look like something dragged through a hedge, take it to a good hairdresser and get them to shape it. Charles Worthington's salons, and special charities in the USA, for example, are experts at this. One thing to remember, if you buy a wig in a specialist shop, tell them you are having chemo and therefore they must deduct VAT.

You don't always lose hair when undergoing chemo. Sometimes a 'cold cap' can help (there are differing reports about this), or sometimes you don't lose it at first, only to find when you go on to another drug, it starts to fall out.

Today, there are better ways to control side effects, and some lucky people say they don't experience any hair loss. Just remember, chemo is helping you to live, and there are over 50 chemotherapy drugs in common use. After the San Antonio Breast Cancer Symposium in December of 2001, the drugs Adriamycin (now called Doxorubicin) and Taxotere® were recommended as first line chemotherapy for newly diagnosed cases of inflammatory breast cancer. However, new drugs are coming along all the time, and you may well be treated by a drug that wasn't even approved when I was writing this.

Chemo brain

The American Cancer Society have confirmed what those of us who have had chemo have been saying all along – there is a condition called 'chemo brain'. This affects our memory when undergoing cancer treatment. No cures as yet – but at least we have something to blame for memory lapses that we were putting down to old age!

When things get you down, an article in the *Hartford Courant* describes how, when the going gets tough, you might want to look at the YouTube website www.youtube.com/user/uconhuskie to see Jessica Gioia of Newington,

Conneticut, describe her treatment, saying that 'chemo is do-able'. She doesn't pull any punches, but she makes you laugh as she describes what can help – water and exercise, and going out to dinner!

And you won't believe this, but . . .

Recently there have been reports that a tiny minority of travellers have had trouble when crossing some frontiers – their cancer treatment had made their fingerprints temporarily unreadable. Roche has issued a statement saying:

> 'Hand-foot syndrome (HFS) is a known side effect of a number of cancer treatments, including Xeloda® (capecitabine). It can cause redness, tenderness, and possibly peeling of the palms and soles. HFS is manageable and generally occurs with increased cumulative dose and longer treatment duration. As such, the syndrome is already on the label for Xeloda®, along with guidelines to manage the syndrome in those patients who experience it. HFS can be minimized with good patient management. It is normal practice, if the syndrome occurs, to interrupt treatment promptly until the syndrome is resolved or reduced to a very low level. Treatment can then be restarted, at a lower dose if required.
>
> HFS symptoms (peeling of the palms) could possibly lead to fingerprint loss. HFS symptoms are reversible by interrupting Xeloda® treatment. Patient safety is of utmost importance to Roche and the company continues to monitor the safety of all patients receiving Xeloda® treatment. For further information please contact: Roche direct line: +44 (0)1707 366 805.'

So if you are flying to the USA, and you seem to have faint fingerprints, it might be an idea to take a letter from your oncologist.

And finally...

I have just heard from a friend who is undergoing chemo that she has been drinking a new canned drink called Alibi. She says it is sweet, but not cloying, with a lemon and a pomegranate flavour. The thing that really impressed both of us is that the makers are doing something so sensible in Afghanistan. They work with a charity to convert opium fields into pomegranate fields. Apparently the yield gives the farmers a similar income, and for every can of Alibi sold, it provides a similar income to three opium poppies (it takes three to create enough heroin for one injection). So we are drinking this like mad! And she says that being fruity, and less sweet, it is easier to keep down.

Miracle cure?

I am not one to place an enormous amount of credence on this, but am prepared to keep an open mind.

Joanne writes to say:

> 'When they booked me for all that radiotherapy to the brain my doctor said my hair would never grow back fully and when it does grow back it will be in tufts. I went to a chappie who makes these great wigs and told him. He sold me his own mixture – something with potassium in. When the treatments were finished, I put this stuff on my bald head and hey presto I have a full thick head of hair.'

This might be worth discussing with a doctor or nurse.

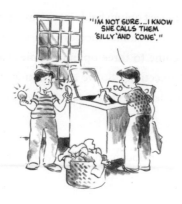

"I'M NOT SURE...I KNOW SHE CALLS THEM 'SILLY 'AND 'CONE'."

Chapter 5

Surgery

Generally, surgery will be scheduled after chemo finishes. Breast cancer surgery is done to prevent cancer recurrence. The idea is to remove the tumour so that it won't reappear in your breast or spread to other parts of your body. You may have several choices for breast surgery, depending on the size of the tumour and other factors. Your surgeon will discuss these with you – and should go over the options carefully. Ask if you don't understand anything, and if you want to know. I didn't – I just wanted them to get on with it, but I am weird like that! Ask your medics if and what you want to know before they go any further.

At this stage, you will probably have been given a bewildering amount of information. You may need to re-read all the literature, but hopefully it is starting to make sense. And you can now talk 'medic-speak' with the best of them!

So what is surgery?

Breast cancer surgery comes in two forms. A mastectomy, which is a complete removal of a breast, or a lumpectomy, removal of part of the breast.

Here is what the cancer charity Macmillan says about surgery:

'[Surgery] means treating illness by removing body tissue. It is one of the main treatments for cancer. Cancer surgery can be used for a number of purposes:

Treatment

Where possible, surgery is used to remove the tumour and nearby tissues that might contain cancer cells. If the cancer has spread to other parts of the body that cannot be totally removed by surgery, you may still have surgery to remove the primary tumour of the initial cancer.

Staging

This is the process that doctors use to work out the size of the cancer and whether it has spread to other parts of the body. Staging can be done at the same time as surgery to remove a tumour. Information about the stage of the cancer is used in planning treatment.

Reconstruction

Surgery can be used to restore:

- a part of the body
- appearance, such as breast reconstruction after a mastectomy.

Risk-reducing

Surgery is sometimes used to remove a part of the body that has a significant risk of developing cancer. This is called risk-reducing or prophylactic surgery. For example, a woman may have surgery to remove her breast tissue because she has a very strong family history of breast cancer.

Palliation

If the cancer cannot be completely removed or cured, surgery can sometimes still help by removing a tumour to reduce its effects, such as blockage, discomfort, or other complications.

If your cancer has spread by the time you are diagnosed, then you may not be offered surgery as your main treatment, because surgery alone will not cure you.

Breast surgery used to leave you with horrendous scars. Today, surgeons will work with you to give you the best and most attractive option possible. Looking down at myself now, you wouldn't even notice my boob was cut away. Even if you have to have a complete mastectomy, this can be much less distressing than in the past.

Reconstruction or breast prosthesis

At the same time as your surgery is scheduled, your surgeon may, or may not, offer you a breast reconstruction.

The National Institute for Health and Clinical Excellence (NICE) guidelines are that patients should be offered breast reconstruction at the same time as their mastectomy, except in exceptional circumstances. As they put it, *'After receiving results of tests, doctor and patient should discuss therapeutic surgery, including immediate reconstruction.'* This means that surgeons in the UK have to offer you the option of a reconstruction during the operation, if this is feasible, to replace what they are taking away.

And, no, you can't have a trade-off. When Adela realized this was classed as cosmetic surgery, she asked if she could swap a boob job for a face-lift! This didn't go down too well.

However, at a recent NICE conference it was said that when offered immediate reconstruction, only a minor percentage of patients took this up – for various reasons. Only about 20 per cent of British women elect to have surgery and reconstruction at the same time. The others decide to 'wait and see'. This could be because patients feel that there is too much to absorb at once, although apparently there are double the number of take-ups in the south-east coastal region than in the north-east and West Midlands. It is your choice to have something done straight away, or to wait until you want this done later.

If you choose to have a reconstruction, you will get implants – silicone forms that go inside your body (in some countries they are called an internal prosthesis, which can be confusing). They are translucent and totally hidden by your own skin. A free DVD called *Breast Reconstruction for Life* includes an introduction, a diary of a typical reconstruction, the procedure from the patient's and the specialist's perspective, and details what finishing touches are available. For a copy go to www.breastreconstructionforlife.org.uk.

If you choose not to have an immediate reconstruction, you can have a breast prosthesis, which is an artificial breast that fits inside a bra to replace all or part of a natural breast. Most breast prostheses are made from soft silicone gel, encased in a thin film, moulded to form the natural shape of a woman's breast, or part of a breast. The outer surface feels soft and smooth, and sometimes may include a nipple outline. This may be supplied separately. The surface that rests against the skin varies, and you can choose one that feels most comfortable for you. You will find more about this in chapter 6.

Before you go into hospital

It may sound silly, but have your exit strategy planned BEFORE you go in to hospital. You will need support when you return home. See chapters 6 and 13 for the type of help you may need and make sure you have a plan arranged beforehand. It will be too late to sort something out when you get home and realize that you are not going to be able to look after the children, lift them up, or even make yourself a cup of tea after surgery.

Going in to hospital

The hospital will tell you what to bring with you, or you can go on to their website to find out.

Although generally one isn't supposed to do this, I suggest taking a pillow with a clean, boiled pillowcase in a separate plastic cover, which you can use when you are in hospital. Those hard plastic hospital pillows are enough to give you bad neck ache. It is strictly against the rules, but . . .

If you have arthritis, polio, or find it difficult to sleep on a hard bed, ask the hospital for an air bed before you go in. Hospitals will try and tell you that a rubber mattress on top of a wooden bed base is good for your back. Phooey!

Anaesthetic

Probably the evening before, or when you arrive in the morning, you will meet your anaesthetist. They are highly trained, and to my mind as important as the surgeon. If you have breathing difficulties, make certain that everyone knows you have to have special treatment. Don't assume that doctors know everything about every disease. Valerie says:

'I had polio as a child and mentioned this to my anaesthetist, who came from a well-known cancer hospital. As there are well over 120,000 ex-polio patients known to still be around, I thought this would be taken into account.

However, afterwards I discovered polio patients can't tolerate the drugs so well. I woke up early in the recovery room, totally on my own and frightened. Because I hadn't been kept warm, it took ages for me to warm up again, and my breathing was shot to pieces. It was two months before I recovered properly.'

So if you have breathing difficulties, make sure you have discussed this fully. If the anaesthetist brushes it off, ask your surgeon to intervene. You have the right to the best possible care whilst you are in the theatre.

Incidentally, what Valerie experienced should never have happened. The Director of Professional Standards at The Royal College of Anaesthetists, Mr Charlie McLaughlan, says, *'there will always be a healthcare professional by the patient's side when they awake from an anaesthetic; this will be either the anaesthetist or a specially trained nurse and often it is both.'*

Personal pills and tablets

You are always told to hand over any drugs or other medication you bring in to hospital with you, but there have been instances of diabetics not being given correct doses. One friend who has to take transplant drugs always hides these in her bag: she knows her local hospital doesn't issue these drugs until the day after patients are admitted – well past the crucial time she has to take them. So hand them over AFTER you know you are going to receive the correct dose at the necessary time.

Valerie says there are good anaesthetists:

'I had heart problems, and was very worried, until my surgeon introduced me to Dr Hunter, the anaesthetist, who was brilliant. He contacted me before my operation to get the name of my polio

specialist. He phoned him to discuss what he was going to do beforehand. My surgeon, Mr Petrou, spent a long time also making sure that I was going to be well looked after, and I was much happier even before I went down to theatre. After a seven-hour operation I felt fantastic! No problems recovering!'

The day of your surgery

You may go into hospital the night before, or on the day of the surgery. This depends on how extensive the operation will be. Here are some tips:

- Let the staff know if you have any allergies. These should be written in large legible writing on your note folder.
- Don't get annoyed with constantly being asked for your name and date of birth. This is a vitally important check that all good nursing and medical staff should carry out EACH time they start a procedure. It is a safeguard for you.
- If your operation is delayed because of problems building up in the operating theatre, you have the right to be kept informed.
- If you are diabetic, it is very important to discuss this with your anaesthetist beforehand, to ensure that any drips that they give you won't send your blood sugar level sky high.
- If you have had polio, or any respiratory disease, the anaesthetist MUST discuss this with you beforehand, as you will need slightly different treatment.
- If you need life-preserving medicine (such as anti-rejection drugs for transplants), make sure you are given hospital replacements BEFORE surrendering yours to ward staff.
- Don't bother to do your nails before you go in to hospital! You will have to remove nail varnish from fingers and toes, so the anaesthetist can check on their colour – a good health indicator.

The operation

When your time comes, things happen very quickly. Before you know it, you are on your way to the theatre. Nice, friendly people welcome you, ask for your arm, start to tell you what is going to happen, but you probably will be off in a dream before they finish the first sentence.

If you are worried about dying on the operating table, it will reassure you to know the statistics. In Britain, there are about five deaths for every million anaesthetics, mostly occurring in patients who are already very unwell and needing emergency treatment.

And when you do wake up, you probably won't feel any different. Most people worry that it will hurt when they wake up. The answer to that is, almost certainly, NO. Today's painkillers are very efficient. My nurse told me about her mother who had been given a morphine drip and thought she was skateboarding down London's fashionable King's Road! Another friend said he could recall every film he had ever seen, and could see each one played out on the hospital wall in glorious Technicolor!

When I was awake enough to get down to enjoying my hallucinations, the drip was taken away because I didn't need it any more. Spoilsports.

So, generally you will be happy, and will drift off to sleep again. With any luck the staff will leave you alone to rest. Do have a good sleep, because once you wake up they will be at you to exercise your arm, get you walking, get you sitting up – they won't leave you in peace! And you will be surprised how quickly you recover. There are seldom complications.

How long will I stay in?

The amount of time you will spend in hospital very much depends on what you and your surgeon have decided on having done. You may only spend a night in – or it could be several days. If you have a mastectomy, you are usually in for five days; seven days for reconstruction.

What usually happens is that the hospital will want to send you home as soon as possible, to avoid the risk of you catching infection in hospital. If you have medical insurance, the company will want you to go home quickly so their payout will be as little as possible.

Recently, the Department of Health announced they were working on discharging patients earlier from hospital. It may save money, but it is bound to cause problems. One of the nurses on a cancer charity helpline said, '*We will get even more calls from people sent home early with no support at home.'* And over-worked mums will have less chance of recovering quickly.

If you do feel fine and are raring to go home, that's wonderful. Take full advantage, but don't overdo it. However, if you dread the thought of having to drag yourself around doing chores at home, just say you are not ready. You deserve the best chance of recovering quickly, and a quiet night on your own can often be the best way.

Phones and TV

You will want to phone friends and family to reassure them. Recently hospitals in UK have given franchises to companies that have come in with incredibly expensive phones. You pay 10p per minute to phone out, but friends are charged 50p per minute to phone you. So most hospitals now allow mobile phones, and you should be able to plug in a charger on the ward. However, long, chatty calls should be made outside the corridor. Other patients may want to sleep.

TV is often charged at an hourly, daily or weekly rate (at the time of writing it was approximately £3.50 per evening).

Do remember that hospitals are open places, and that thieves know patients are easy to rob. So leave jewellery and large amounts of money at home.

Single-sex wards

Luckily, cancer patients in Britain are more likely to be nursed in a completely single-sex ward. However, if you do find that you are in a bay next door to others of the opposite sex, according to the Department of Health, you are perfectly entitled to ask to be moved.

Teeth

If your teeth are loose after the operation, it might be because the breathing tubes were not inserted correctly. This shouldn't happen, but if a tooth wobbles, draw it to the ward sister's attention immediately. If you wait until you get home, the hospital will say it didn't happen whilst you were under their care – they don't want to pay out for a repair that can cost £1,000.

Side effects

Whilst in the hospital, it is important that you let the doctor or nurse know if you have side effects. Don't just think they will go away. Chances are whatever is bothering you *won't*. And when you return home it is too late to suddenly think, *'Whom can I ask?'* Ask while you are in hospital, when the team is still available – even if they are rushed off their feet. You have a problem and you need attention.

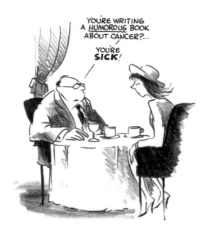

Chapter 6
After your operation

You will feel tired. You just don't realize how tired – but ask anyone who has had this operation, and they all say, 'I didn't realize how it would hit me.' You will probably be even more tired than most breast cancer patients, as more than likely you will have had treatment such as chemo before surgery – so building up even more fatigue. I just thought I would hit you with the bad news first!

Added to the fatigue, you will almost certainly have none or limited movement in the arm next to the operation site, which means cooking, housework or even a cup of tea is going to be a problem. You go home, wander around trying to tell yourself the operation is over, and can't understand why you feel 'out of it' and tired.

There are some people who bounce around saying they feel fine, but eventually it will hit them too – days or even weeks later. Doctors are finally realizing that fatigue is a big factor in recovery, so tell yourself that your body is telling you what it can and can't do. Listen to it, and look after it. If you have young kids, they won't be able to understand why you can't lift them up when they want a cuddle, but this will be totally impossible for several days. If you can, hide under the bedclothes for as many days as it takes.

Taking care of your wound after breast surgery

The following information is taken from www.healthline.com (an American website). It has some clear advice:

> 'After breast cancer surgery, you will have a bandage or a dressing over the place where you had surgery. You may also have tubes in your breast to remove blood and lymph fluids that build up during the healing process. This means you will have to drain the tubes, measure the fluid, and learn to identify any problems you may need to tell your doctor or nurse about. The nurses will show you what you have to do.

This site is much more honest than the NHS, which says:

> 'Some women feel fine within a month. Others need a few more weeks. Take as much time as you need to adjust to the changes in your life and body.'

I found that the dressing was genuinely waterproof, so I was able to have a gentle bath the day after surgery, but I would suggest leaving the power shower until the dressing is off!

After surgery, your body needs time to recover. You will receive information about helping your body to heal. You may also be given a temporary prosthesis to wear during this time. And you'll learn what complications to watch for.

As you recover from the surgery, your doctor will tell you when it is safe to begin exercising. Generally you will be visited by a breast care nurse or physiotherapist whilst you are in hospital, who give you exercises to do. Make sure you do them, as these help recovery. Your goal will be to regain normal range of motion and use of your arm.

Breast prostheses

Breast Cancer Care has a short video on its website, featuring Wendy Morgan, who has been living with a breast prosthesis for nearly four decades (www. breastcancercare.org.uk and click on 'Treatment', then 'Surgery', then 'Breast

Prostheses'). They say that in the first weeks after surgery, your chest can be sensitive, so wearing silicone prosthesis can be uncomfortable until your chest has healed – about six to eight weeks.

During these weeks you should be given a light fabric-covered prosthesis known as a 'softie' or a 'cumfie'. You may find that the softie rides up because it is so light. It may look better if you adjust the stuffing and either pin or stitch it to the bottom of your bra cup.

You will need a very soft, stretchy bra in which to insert your softie. This may be one you already own, but it needs to be easy to put on because your shoulder may be stiff at first. Your breast care nurse in hospital should have given you exercises to help ease this stiffness.

Once your chest area is fully healed, you will need a well-fitting, supportive bra to be successfully fitted with your permanent prosthesis. This is so that your prosthesis matches the shape and size of your natural breast, and is held comfortably and securely in place. If it doesn't fit well, others will tell you of hilarious or humiliating occasions when their prosthesis popped out.

You can choose from many different types. Some are filled with foam or liquid silicone. Some are self-adhering. They are made to move, feel, and weigh similar to a normal breast. A prosthesis not only allows you to appear as you did before your surgery, it also helps balance the weight in your chest. This may help prevent neck or back pain if you have large breasts. Insurance pays for most prostheses if you have a prescription or letter demonstrating medical necessity.

The dark and light of it

Finding a prosthesis that matches your skin colour could be traumatic. Marina Raime of Betterdays cancer care (www.betterdays.uk.com) has campaigned for better services, and says:

> 'After undergoing surgery for a bilateral mastectomy, I was shocked and horrified to find that the surgical department suggested I look for a pop sock that matched my skin tone. When I enquired as to the purpose of the pop sock. I was told, "So we can match it to your breast prosthesis." I felt insulted and offended by the suggestion. I later enquired about what the policy on prosthesis was for women

of colour. I was informed, "That is the policy". The policy is due to supply and demand. Due to the lack of black women requesting skin-coloured prosthesis, and the high costs of custom-made breast forms, some NHS Trusts fail to provide or even stock skin-coloured breasts for women of colour to view at their prosthesis (breast) fitting.

After carrying out further enquiries, I discovered that coloured swatches are available, and they come in various shades of browns. It is my understanding that it's the breast clinic's duty to make sure these swatches are available. In addition breast forms should be available for women of colour to view on appointment. If that's not evidence of inequality and cultural insensitivity in service provision then I don't know what is.

For me as a young woman it's all about confidence. That's why black women need prostheses that complement their skin colour. I want to wear them for sports, running, swimming, dancing, without fear and embarrassment. Betterdays has campaigned to help trusts find your shade.'

Marina's work seems to have had results; asking Trusts today what their policy is, there seems much more awareness and willingness to help.

Post-operative treatment

Successful treatment of your cancer is the first step towards a healthy future. Now you can begin a lifelong follow-up programme, which should include visits to your healthcare provider, mammograms, and breast self-exams. Maintaining each part of this programme will help to give you peace of mind as you begin your life after treatment.

Lymphoedema

After breast surgery, fluid may collect and cause swelling in the arm on the side of your surgery. This is called lymphoedema (or lymphodema). It occurs when lymph nodes under the arm are removed or the under-arm area is treated with radiation therapy, causing the normal flow of fluids in the arm to be reduced.

You should be given written advice on how to avoid this.

Lymphoedema can occur right after surgery, or months or years later. So, if your arm becomes swollen, hot or painful, call your doctor straight away.

Lymphoedema may last fewer than six months (called acute lymphoedema) or longer than six months (called chronic lymphoedema). It can be a temporary side effect of the surgery or the condition could be triggered by an injury or strain to your arm – some even say an insect bite. To reduce your risk, avoid heavy lifting and protect your arm from injury. And have injections and blood pressure collars fitted on the opposite arm, not the one nearest the affected breast.

If treated, swelling from lymphoedema can be managed. If not, swelling can become severe. Treatment includes specialized massage using the Vodder method. In Britain, many treatment clinics have closed down, but the Lymphoedema Support Network can help. For more information, go to www.lymphoedema.org or call 020 7351 4480.

Christina wrote to her MEP and got him to approach her Primary Care Trust to approve payment in a private clinic. You can find out more on my site, www.after-cancer.com/lymphoedema.

Reconstructive surgery

The decision to have reconstructive breast surgery is very personal. Everyone has different ideas. Don't be forced into making a snap decision. Many take weeks or even months to decide. It is entirely up to you, and depends a lot on how you think you will feel after a mastectomy. If you think you would feel uncomfortable with a flat chest or wearing a prosthesis, you may want to consider reconstructive surgery. If you don't mind how you'll look or don't want to have any extra surgery, you may not want to do it.

Reconstructive surgery can be done at the time of your mastectomy, or you can schedule it for a later date. You may need more than one operation to complete the reconstruction. The aim is to match the remaining natural breast.

What happens during reconstructive surgery depends on the type of surgery you decide to have. You can opt for reconstructive surgery using artificial implants, or you can choose to have surgery that rebuilds your breast using tissue, such as skin, fat, and sometimes muscle, from another part of your body. A combination of these techniques is used for some women.

Our breasts are very personal to us, so it is not surprising that we find it difficult to think about this. However, about half of all women who have a mastectomy choose to have breast reconstruction, either at the time of their initial surgery or afterwards. Your surgeon can help you decide whether to have reconstructive surgery. You will be advised to wait if during or after the operation is not the best time for you. It will depend on:

- how much of the breast tissue has been removed
- how healthy the tissue is at the planned operation site
- whether or not you have had radiotherapy to the breast area or chest wall
- your general health and body build
- your personal preference

It is possible to create a new nipple, which can be done as a separate operation once the reconstructed breast has settled into its final shape. It may be possible for it to be done at the same time as the breast reconstruction. Not everyone chooses to have a nipple.

Macmillan has very helpful information about the different types of surgery and procedures on their website, www.macmillan.org.uk. It is worth looking at this, as reconstruction techniques are updated all the time.

Micropigmentation

Teresa Frake, Training Manager of Beauty Concepts International Ltd, says:

'When ladies have had the breast reconstructed, the breasts don't always look absolutely even, depending on how many operations they have had to go through. The areola (the area around the nipple) and the nipple are sometimes removed completely, and if it is a total reconstruction then the breast is just left 'plain'.

With micropigmentation, which is a form of tattooing, the area can look more like a regular breast and goes a long way to improving self-confidence. The areola is tattooed on and a nipple can be tattooed also. The pigmented area usually lasts about two years or sometimes even longer and may just need a top up after this time.'

Go to www.beautyconcepts.co.uk or call 01273 837302 for more information.

How do I say 'Thank you'?

When you leave hospital, hopefully you will take many happy memories of kindness and helpfulness shown by staff. You may want to say thank you. No one will expect a present, or think any less of you if you can't afford one.

Annie says:

'I was treated at a private hospital, because my Trust sent me there. There were lots of patients from all over the world giving watches and other gifts. I just went round with thank-you cards, and the nurses were just as appreciative. Nurses have a pretty good idea if you haven't much money, and they appreciate the thought.'

Tina says:

'My therapy was to bake cakes! After running a business no one could imagine me with apron and mixing bowl – but as I beat the eggs I was getting rid of frustrations! I did apologize, as I knew staff were always on diets, but the nurses, radiographers, physio etc. ate up my cakes with enthusiasm.'

I asked one of my nurses what they liked to receive. *'This is a very sticky area in so much as we are constrained by the NMC (Nursing and Midwifery Council) guidelines as to what we can receive as a gift. It is very difficult to suggest what one "should" give the nurses. As you correctly state, most nurses are on diets!'*

A straw poll among fellow patients has come up with these ideas:

- **Surgeon** Write a thank-you letter and send it to him/her at hospital
- **Anaesthetist** We always forget that this person is just as important as the surgeon. They do appreciate a letter.
- **Ward Sister** A thank-you card addressed to the sister but you could ask for your thanks to be passed on to the rest of the staff.
- **Nurses** Check before you buy chocolates that your nurses would be glad

to receive them! If you are strapped for cash, write thank-you notes for each nurse. One friend worked for a PR company. She went round the company cupboards, filled a big straw basket with samples ranging from cosmetics to T-shirts. She was very popular when she delivered it to the nurses.

- **Your favourite nurse** A card saying how much you appreciated what she did for you. And if you have the cash, get something special for her – from nice hand cream to a voucher for the local spa.
- **Cleaners** Possibly chocolates for them. They don't need to diet with all that sweeping!

The staff work very hard and really appreciate someone who takes the time to write a note.

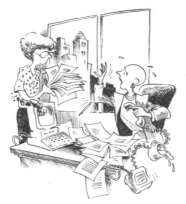

"NOT NOW... I'M HAVING A NO HAIR DAY!"

Chapter 7
Radiotherapy

Radiotherapy is the use of high energy X-rays and similar rays (such as electrons) to treat disease. Since the discovery of X-rays, radiation has been used more and more in medicine, both to help with diagnosis (by taking pictures with X-rays), and as a treatment (radiotherapy). As Macmillan says, while radiation obviously has to be used very carefully, doctors and radiographers have a lot of experience in its use in medicine.

According to NHS Choices, radiotherapy is the safe use of controlled doses of radiation to treat disease, especially cancer. Radiotherapy has been used since 1895, but we are still learning. The latest treatments can involve giving larger but fewer doses. There is on-going research into the value of this, as well as giving treatment during your operation to cut down on sessions later on.

How it works
Radiotherapy destroys the cancer cells in the treated area. Although normal cells are also affected, they are better at repairing themselves.

The treatment consists of pointing an X-ray machine at the part of the body to be treated. This machine will 'deliver' a measured dose of radiotherapy rays directed at your tumour.

Cancer Research UK says:

> 'A course of radiotherapy is usually given over a number of days or weeks. Each treatment is known as a "fraction", and is usually given Monday to Friday, with a rest at weekends to help normal cells recover.'

Your clinical oncologist will supervise, plan and monitor treatment carefully. You will have regular appointments during your treatment course to ensure everything is going smoothly.

Planning or mapping

If you have surgery before radiotherapy, the radiotherapy team will call you in for a meeting to plan your treatment course as soon as the swelling goes down. During the session, they take accurate measurements of the area to be treated, and build a cast or support to help you stay still whilst undergoing treatment. They will probably tattoo a few minute dots on your body to help them align your body precisely when having treatment. This doesn't hurt, and I could never find them, but the team know what to look for.

You may have a CT (computerized tomography) scan of the area to be treated. This takes many images from different angles to build up a 3-D picture.

The radiographers take lots and lots of measurements, which are fed into the computer to enable the machine to target precisely the area to be treated.

This whole session generally takes over an hour, so you may need pain relief if it hurts to lie on a hard bed.

What happens during treatment?

You may have to travel a long way for treatment, which can be inconvenient. However, the equipment costs millions, and you want to be treated by the most up-to-date machines, so you may have to put up with long travelling times.

In Britain, you can apply for help with paying car parking and road congestion charges. Some road bridge authorities will also wave their charges. Ask for forms at the PALS office (Patient Advice and Liaison Office) in every hospital, or from any Macmillan nurse.

Setting up

Every day during treatment, the radiographers will be very busy at the start of each session, setting you up precisely so that the machine can aim directly at the target area. Then they leave the room, leaving you all on your own. This is so that they can start your session as quickly as possible, as they have to fit in so many patients, but it can feel as if they are abandoning you!

The machine is massive, and it generally moves above you. The noise and the movement can be unsettling, but it won't drop on you – it's far too valuable!

Radiotherapy suites are changing enormously, but there are still some that are old-fashioned. If yours is gloomy, it's as well to remember that you are being given life-enhancing treatment.

Adela says:

'During my treatment, I felt I was on an impersonal conveyor belt. The hospital used the patient changing room for storing goods, and we had to undress in the treatment rooms – open to all and sundry to walk in. One day I exploded – there wasn't even a hook to hang my clothes. The next day they had put up a hook, six foot high and out of reach.'

Luckily this type of treatment suite is being phased out. At Parkside Hospital in Wimbledon, the rooms are painted in happy colours, and each patient is provided with a gown for their sole use during treatment.

Carol Hurd, Parkside's Radiotherapy Manager, says:

'We always strive to make the department as patient-friendly as possible. For that reason we have, in the last year, had a TV and a coffee machine put in the waiting area and aim to ensure that the reception desk is manned most of the time so patients feel welcomed, and are able to ask questions prior to their being called for treatment. We have also installed a suggestions box, although we're unable to comply with one patient's suggestion that we have a puppy in the department!'

At a recent postgraduate course for radiographers at Kingston University, some of the participants said their departments held welcome meetings at the start of every treatment cycle to explain what was going to happen during the four to six-week course. Patients could meet staff, ask them questions and would feel at home when they came in.

How you will feel during treatment

You can't explain why – after all, you are just lying down for ten minutes each day – but you can feel very tired. My unscientific explanation for this is that your body is beavering away inside, repairing the healthy cells that have got zapped, along with the damaged ones.

You may want to go to bed for a short sleep when you return home, especially towards the end of your treatment.

Burns

Your breast will probably start to burn, unless you do something about it. I was told to use aloe vera gel (make sure it is the 98 per cent pure one) and I slapped this on four times a day. My breast didn't burn at all, even though my surgeon told me two years later that the treatment site was still warm.

Some hospitals won't tell you about aloe vera – or will suggest other creams. Michaela says: '*I got horrid burns, and the technician suggested some cream or other – with the comment, "It probably won't do any good." It didn't.*' So she tried Equilibria, an aloe vera gel from Italy, and as she spread it on, the burn visibly lost its angry colour and calmed down. Equilibria is currently undergoing clinical trials. My hospital sold a similar product at £12.50 a tube, but the same size Equilibria tube from the chemist is half this price.

If you are told you can't use deodorants, mention that French hospitals now use one made by Evolife. And if you develop burns, again this company has come up with Evoskin, a range of products that calms and soothes, including a spray so you don't need to rub it in. More about this company and their products on page 138.

Body hair

The hair will fall out around the treatment area; not on your head or as drastically as during chemo.

Interim meeting

About halfway through your course you will probably be called back, and the team will measure you and check X-rays and scans, to ensure things haven't moved and you are being targeted in the right place.

Medical notes

You should know where the record of your treatment is kept, as all the doses are recorded carefully. Specialists will need to refer to these notes should you ever need more radiotherapy, for cancer or any other disease.

And that's it!

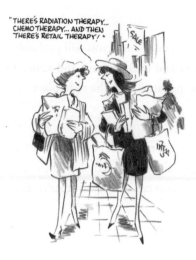

"THERE'S RADIATION THERAPY...
CHEMO THERAPY... AND THEN
THERE'S RETAIL THERAPY!"

Chapter 8

Hormonal drugs

As well as the drugs you will be given during chemotherapy, you will probably be put on hormonal drugs. These are generally given as pills, although some come as a monthly or periodic injection. You will probably be on these for several years.

Go on the internet and you will be able to find the clinical trials data for your particular hormonal drug. It is a happy exercise, as you can see how rates of survival are improving every year, and much of the improvement is thanks to these drugs. However, there is a sting in the tail: side effects can be very nasty. It is reckoned:

- 5 per cent of us will have no side effects
- 95 per cent of us will have side effects

I hope you are among the 5 per cent. Hopefully your doctor will talk you through possible side effects, but if he or she doesn't have the time, the next chapter goes into these in more detail. And if, like me, you end up with the short straw, keep reminding yourself that these pills are helping to give you a better future and a longer life.

Drugs

Probably the best-known hormonal drug is tamoxifen. Others you might be offered are Aromasin®, Arimidex®, letrozole and Herceptin®, but watch the media as new ones are being developed every day. Much of the following information has been taken from copy supplied by the drug manufacturers.

Tamoxifen

Currently, this is probably the most prescribed drug. It is often the first drug you are given (the others come later). The way tamoxifen works is complicated but its main function is as an anti-oestrogen drug. Oestrogen (also known as estrogen) is a general term for the primary female sex hormone and used in oral contraceptives. Most breast cancers need supplies of oestrogen to grow. Cancer cells have proteins called receptors on their surface to which the sex hormones attach. Cancers with oestrogen-receptors on the surface of their cells are called 'oestrogen-receptor-positive' (ER-positive) and tamoxifen is most effective against these cancers. Under normal circumstances, when oestrogen comes into contact with the receptors, it fits into them and activates the cancer cells to divide so that the tumour grows. Tamoxifen imitates the action of oestrogen and fits into the receptor but does not activate cell division. The tamoxifen stays in place so the cancer cells either grow more slowly or stop growing altogether. Tamoxifen can greatly reduce the chance of ER-positive cancers coming back after surgery. It can also be used to shrink large tumours down before surgery so that they can be removed.

The side effects can be so bad that many patients come off these. PLEASE DON'T. If the pills make you feel like this, turn to the next chapter, where there is a whole lot of information gathered from France, Germany and USA on clinically approved products that can help.

Aromasin® (exemestane)

This is one of the aromatase inhibitors – a new generation of wonder drugs. It works by preventing the action of an enzyme in the body called the aromatase enzyme – the female sex hormone oestrogen – in women who have gone through the menopause. Most breast cancers are sensitive to oestrogen, and their growth is encouraged by this hormone. So the theory is, block it off and you starve the breast cancer cells. This stops them from growing.

It is generally prescribed after a preliminary two or three years on tamoxifen.

If you are put on this drug, your doctor should carefully monitor your bone density, as this drug can cause you to develop osteoporosis. And don't take it if you are fructose intolerant.

Arimidex® (anastrozole)

This is an aromatase inhibitor, and works in a similar way to Aromasin®. Most of the side effects are similar, except this can also cause carpal tunnel syndrome. This is when you get numbness in your hands and fingers. When I got this, the consultant looking after me had no idea it was caused by Arimidex® – I found this out ages afterwards on the internet.

Herceptin® (trastuzumab)

Hailed as a miracle drug when it first came out, what the media didn't mention is that it is only suitable for a very small percentage of cancers; those that are HER2-positive. It is considered an immune therapy, as it imitates the way the body's own immune system fights cancer. If suitable for this, you will be given Herceptin® as an infusion (dripped into your body via a needle inserted into a vein). The first dose can bring up flu-like symptoms, but generally side effects lessen with each treatment.

In early trials there was some risk to the heart, but now doctors monitor the drug more closely, and are more careful about the cocktail of drugs that is administered during treatment.

letrozole (Femara®)

You must be particularly careful if you have liver problems or drug allergies, and limit alcohol intake as this might increase side effects.

Other drugs – particularly painkillers – can play havoc with your skin. Just expect side effects, and realize they are part and parcel of the treatment. When taking these drugs, drink lots of water, and give your skin extra attention. See the next chapter and my 'hero products' in Chapter 19 for help and recommendations.

Prevention

When enquiring medical minds get together, things come out of meetings that can be of real benefit to us. At a recent oncologists' meeting in Paris, several mentioned that they were working on preventing side effects on the skin by giving patients products to prevent side effects *before* they presented with them. Technically, they were there to talk about acne, lesions, cracked skin, oncholysis (nail trauma) and highly sensitive skin or mucous membranes that sometimes cause us trouble. They admitted this question concerning quality of life for cancer patients can be taboo. Many doctors try to brush away these symptoms, and patients feel they can't complain in case they are considered vain, or – even worse – have to put up with them. As one expert said, *'current treatments used to address these issues today are far from satisfactory; often the solution is to reduce dosage or break up the treatment schedule'.*

In France, over one million people are treated for cancer every year; probably more than two-thirds will suffer side effects to their skin. In 2006, a brilliant young dermatologist, Dr Geraldine Reynaert, had been working with patients suffering from skin diseases of neurological origin. She then began working with cancer patients, and discovered the products also worked with our problems. She had used products from a firm called Evolife, and they were as excited as she was that there was a new use to help patients. Together they started to work out which products in their lithium-based range would be of benefit. Oncologists around France were alerted, and started to use the products. For more information about Evolife, go to page 138.

The French have 'Cancer Strategy Plans', but unlike ours, they get on with practical ways of implementing them. They now have the best post-cancer survival rates. In France, the doctors will listen to your problem, then ring straight through to an oncologist to discuss what can be done. So simple, and so helpful.

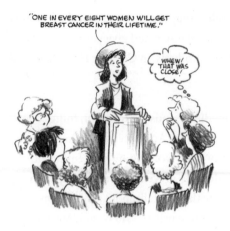

Chapter 9

Handling side effects

When you start taking those tiny little hormonal drug pills, you might discover that you and the medical profession are speaking a different language. In my experience, you ask about the side effects you are experiencing – something nasty like peeling skin or losing sight in an eye – and your oncologist looks at you and says, 'I've never heard of that before. I don't know what to suggest.' But it's their job to *know* what to advise, and if not, to send you to someone else who can help. So it is up to you to be assertive and persistent. Don't be fobbed off. And if you can't find a solution, don't despair. This chapter is all about dealing with possible side effects, from simple problems to big ones such as peeling skin, loss of sight, 'brillo pad' face or losing nails. Helping with these side effects is not rocket science. It is plain common sense allied to good background knowledge. Something that other countries offer, but our NHS often doesn't have the time or funds for.

At a recent NICE press conference, the eminent professors were lined up to speak on NICE's plans for breast cancer care in the future. Sitting at either end were two patients, invited on to the working party. When the chairman turned to the two patients for their comments, they didn't repeat all the golden promises for the future. Instead, both highlighted how they felt they had been abandoned after their treatment finished in hospital; how they felt alone, unable to find information or help. Afterwards, they were swamped by the TV crews, who recognized a genuine need.

In defence of the medics, every patient reacts differently and every patient will have a different combination of side effects. If you are lucky, you will sail through treatment without any problems, but if not, don't despair.

- Talk to others and find out what has worked for them.
- Read information below from patients who have found solutions.
- Keep on and on at your oncologist.
- Go on the web – you could try my website www.after-cancer.com, which is written by patients, not by medically-qualified people, but is careful to only mention products that have had clinical trials, or been approved by cancer charities or various Food and Drug Agencies.
- Don't take any herbal supplements, Chinese medicines, extra vitamins, without asking your doctor. Even the most innocuous herb can react violently with the chemicals in drugs, so check this out. If people say it worked for them, you might be taking a different combination of drugs, or have different physical symptoms.

Statistics

A recent NHS survey said over 50 per cent of patients came off hormonal drugs because they couldn't stand side effects. Another survey in Ireland reported that a significant percentage of those who came off these drugs had a recurrence of their cancer. So it is in your interest to learn how to stay on the drugs.

Researchers led by Cancer Research UK's Professor Jack Cuzick have found that these side effects are actually a good sign that the treatment is working. The scientists analysed data from a trial called ATAC (anastrozole, tamoxifen as adjuvant treatment), which compared tamoxifen with anastrozole for post-menopausal women with breast cancer. The study showed that, although both drugs can effectively treat the disease, the cancer was around 25 per cent less likely to return in those who had taken anastrozole. In this new research, published in the journal *Lancet Oncology*, the scientists looked at around 2,000 women taking each drug, and studied those who had hot flushes or joint pain within three months of starting the trial. They found that women with hot flushes were 16 per cent less likely to have a recurrence. Those with joint pain were 40 per cent less likely to have the cancer come back, whilst the lowest rates of recurrence were seen in women with both side effects.

Cancer Research UK says it shows that side effects can be a good indication that treatment is working – at least in this situation – and that women who experience them should be encouraged to stick with the treatment. But there are a few other things to bear in mind. Firstly, this finding does not show that women who don't experience side effects will not get any benefit from their treatment. Less than half of the patients in the ATAC trial had hot flushes on either drug, while between 20 and 30 per cent had joint pain. But both drugs are highly effective in the majority of patients – the cancer came back in only 12 per cent of women on anastrozole, and 16 per cent on tamoxifen.

This tells us that if you don't have side effects from treatment, your chances of avoiding recurrence are very good. But if you do have them, your chances may be better. **It is up to you to find things that can help with side effects, and stay on the drugs.**

Anti-depressants

The respected news agency *Bloomberg* recently reported that tamoxifen is less effective when taken with anti-depressants such as Paxil, Prozac or Zoloft. Indeed, tumours were more than twice as likely to return as those on tamoxifen alone. Doctors started treating hot flushes with anti-depressants after a US study linked the former standard remedy, hormone replacement therapy, to an increased risk of breast cancer and heart attacks. However, the research, by Medco Health Solutions Inc, showed that other types of anti-depressants, such as Effexor, may be safer for women on tamoxifen. Powel Brown, Director of Cancer Prevention at the Lester and Sue Smith Breast Cancer Center in the United States said that, *'Effexor doesn't interfere with tamoxifen so that is the preferred drug for oncologists to treat hot flushes. We need to get that message out to primary care doctors and psychiatrists and gynecologists so they will be aware that anti-depressants like Paxil have a risk of inhibiting tamoxifen.'*

Ask your oncologist for the latest update.

Side effects

Cancer Research UK, in its *Science Update*, confirms, 'there is no such thing as a cancer drug without side effects – at least, not a drug that actually works. If a treatment has an effect on a biological process that has gone awry, then it will also affect healthy cells in the body, causing side effects.' So here are some that you might experience and what you can do about them (in alphabetical order).

Carpal tunnel syndrome

This is when your hands become painful, with weakened grip, numbness and tingling. It is caused by pressure on a nerve in your wrist. It is often associated with repetitive strain injury but it can be a side effect of drugs, particularly Arimidex®.

Cramp

If you experience cramp, the advice is:
- stay well hydrated
- take electrolyte replacement (e.g. sodium, potassium, calcium, magnesium) if specific deficiencies are noted
- if diuretics are taken, avoid stimulants like caffeine, and nicotine
- gently stretch muscles before exercising, and before going to bed.

There are many drugs that are said to work on cramp, including Diazepam, but my favourite pharmacist says there are problems with most. You could start by drinking tonic water. It contains quinine , and if this doesn't work, you could try quinine tablets.

Diarrhoea

If you have diarrhoea, the best way of handling this is described in the book, *Even the Eyebrows?* by Sharon Morrison (AuthorHouse, ISBN 978-1-43892334-5). She devised an emergency kit:
- scented nappy sacks
- night-time sanitary towels
- wet wipes

- spare knickers
- Imodium Instant

She also gives a very funny description about this embarrassing side effect, often overlooked by medics.

Fatigue

This is a constant complaint. One way of dealing with it is to take an old-fashioned nap in the middle of the afternoon. Gradually you will probably find that you need naps less and less, until you can go most days without one. But the moment you find you are tired, off to bed!

For more solutions, there is a book written for ME sufferers called *Fighting Fatigue* by Sue Pemberton and Catherine Berry (Hammersmith Press, ISBN 978-1-905140-28-2). They recommend catnaps too, and say not to worry if you can't sleep through the night. As your body has slowed down, you may not need as much sleep as before but, *'quality not quantity also applies to sleep.'*

Another tip is to drink decaffeinated drinks and manage your activity throughout the day – don't do everything all at once! And they make a sensible point: stress is a normal and necessary part of everyday life, so don't worry too much about being over-stressed.

If you are working, sometimes HR departments can be very understanding, finding you a reclining chair in a quiet office to have your nap. Tell them that you will only need 20 to 30 minutes to set you up again.

Hair, hands and nails

We can get what's known as 'straw hair' or painful splitting nails. NailTek® are an American company that makes products especially for cancer patients. Their products were recommended to me by Francesca Manning, the manicurist at the Royal Marsden. If you have splitting skin on your feet, the NHS does supply a product called Flexitol. Your doctor may never have heard of it, but it is available, so do ask. For more information, see Chapter 19 – Hero products.

Hot flushes

These can be embarrassing and severe, with sweat pouring off you. Here are some tips that might help:

- Wear layers of clothing that can be taken off easily.
- If your flushes are caused by tamoxifen, ask if you can split the dose.
- Have a rest during the day – then it doesn't matter if you don't sleep through the night.
- Take walks and other exercise.
- Wear cotton, silk, wool or other natural materials that absorb moisture and don't cling.
- Carry a mini fan around with you!

If you have flushes at night, friends report that the Chillow is a safe, cool and soothing way to ease the discomfort of hot flushes and night sweats. It is exactly what it sounds like – a cool pillow, designed to help with the misery of hot flushes. It is a thin, cushioned pad that lies on top of a normal pillow or inside the pillowcase. It works by taking heat away from the body and keeping you cool throughout the night, helping you to sleep naturally.

It is available from Soothsoft at www.chillow.co.uk or call 08700 117 174.

Itching

Cancer Research UK has useful tips on coping with itching, and the following is an extract:

- Limit the number of baths you take and use lukewarm water with very little or no soap.
- Instead of soap, you can use a moisturizing liquid.
- Pat your skin dry with a towel rather than rubbing.
- Drying the skin thoroughly reduces the chance of chaffing and fungal infection.
- Moisturize your skin straight after you bathe.
- Avoid scented or lanolin-based lotions.
- Use odourless and colourless moisturizer.
- Wear cotton and linen, rather than wool or man-made materials which can irritate the skin.
- Keep your bedclothes light.

- Try to keep an even, cool temperature in your room, as getting hot can make itching worse.
- Drink plenty of fluids – preferably 2 to 3 litres of water a day.
- Keep your nails short to reduce the risk of damaging your skin
- If you want to scratch, it can sometimes help to gently pinch an area of skin close to the itch or to rub, tap or press the area. You could even use an ice bandage, which will have a counter-irritant effect.

Joanna says:

'The biggest side effect I've had and am having is itching skin. It drives me mad. My oncologist said to use baby oil or tissue oil and lots of body butter type creams. I must admit it does help. I changed my diet as well. I don't eat dairy anymore. I've changed to soya. My weight should have gone up on Neophedan but it hasn't and I think it's because I cut out dairy. I try to walk 20 minutes every day as well.'

Baby oil may not work for all itching, but French oncologists say that good gels or creams are probably going to help more people. Contact your doctor or nurse if the itchy area is getting more red and sore, or if there is any pus.

Nausea

Another common side effect. The nurses often have remedies. Drinking tonic water is surprisingly effective for some people. However, recent studies at University of Rochester Medical Center showed *'ginger supplements reduce chemotherapy-related nausea'.* Although they didn't follow through with trials of hormonal drugs, there is a lot of anecdotal evidence to suggest that ginger can be helpful.

Painful joints

A side effect from all hormonal drugs. If not too bad, the old remedy of a long soak in a warm bath and then bed can work well. If the symptoms are worse, ask your doctor to refer you on. There are drugs that can help, but they need careful supervision. Many patients swear by supplements; but again, ask your doctor just in case they contain something that will react with another drug you are taking.

Skin problems

All drugs are bad for your skin. Some are worse than others. Hormonal drugs kill off cells, which include those that make your skin soft and young-looking. Our skin is our largest and most important feature, so it is bound to get the lion's share of side effects. If you get painful, peeling, dry, itching skin, DON'T think you mustn't make a fuss. DON'T even think that you are wasting doctor's time and they will think you are vain. Skin needs looking after, for men and women. All of a sudden you can find you have horrid lines cropping up; open pores; little bits of flaky skin all over your body; peeling nails. It can get worse (sorry!).

There are excellent products out there, that have been clinically trialled and developed to help with skin problems caused by cancer drugs. If you know what to ask for, you can get these products at good chemists, through some good dermatologists or online. See Chapter 19 for more information.

Companies that have had recognized clinical trials include:

- La Roche Posay
- iS Clinical
- Evolife (currently undergoing trials)

Companies with research departments that understand 'drug problem skin' are:

- Clinique
- Estée Lauder
- Dr Bragi
- Sisley

Companies that pride themselves on providing 'natural' products are:

- Barefoot Botanicals
- Weleda
- Cowshed
- Udderly Smooth

People peer anxiously at labelling, worried about additives and preservatives in products. There has been a huge amount of talk about risks associated with parabens, which are present in products from topical dermatological medications to vitamins. You may like to buy completely natural products, but even those have to have preservatives or they will soon go off. My feeling – for what it's worth – is that cancer drugs are so harmful, a few additives aren't going to have a hope of doing worse damage! I believe that you get what you pay for, and good skincare companies look at the benefits to you.

Sonia says:

> 'When I asked companies what they recommended for my skin, quite rightly, none of them would give me anything to help until I could produce a letter from my doctor saying my skin was healed. Once my doctor gave me the go-ahead and said I could tolerate creams, Clinique took over. They make a fabulous Deep Comfort Body Butter, which does exactly what it says on the label. Smoothing that all over my skin three times a day eventually brought my horrible peeling skin under control, and now I only use it once a day.
>
> I did think I should try to see if the NHS could contribute to the cost, and was given several products to try, including Cetraben and Oilatum Cream. They are OK, but sadly not nearly as effective, so it was back to Clinique!'

Clinique are well aware of problems caused by drugs, and they have developed special creams to help patients. They even took stands at dermatology and other medical conferences to tell the medical profession about this, but doctors just weren't interested. They have produced an excellent booklet, written for the medical profession, which lists every ingredient in their recommended range, so staff can check if anything might produce a reaction to certain drugs.

Dr Bragi is a professor and doctor of biochemistry at the University of Iceland, and one of Iceland's top science lecturers. As a result of his work, he has developed a range of products that are very popular with dermatologists and plastic surgeons, due to their healing properties. The enzymes these contain have been extensively tested in strictly supervised clinical trials on different conditions including arthritis, wounds, eczema, psoriasis, rosacea, burns, acne, inflammation, lupus and impetigo. Currently the enzyme is undergoing trials for skin reformation and scarring correction. Dr Bragi products have a different 'feel', and in fact you can't put another cream on top of the face moisturizer for 15 minutes. But it's well worth waiting, as patients say they are extremely good on 'cancer drug' skin.

Evolife is another skincare range, developed in France and currently undergoing testing in French hospitals.

All the companies I mention here make suitable products for black and minority ethnic skins. They say that their consultants can give advice if you need to use any special creams. Anthelios (La Roche Posay) is recommended for people with black skin or those who have vitiligo, and is also recommended for every skin type that is photosensitive or photosensitive as a consequence of photosensitizing drugs (chemotherapeutic drugs are known photosensitizers).

I find it strange that none of the hospitals or charities in Britain sell good skincare. Most major cancer hospitals in the US have a shop selling approved skincare, so patients and their friends can buy helpful products that add benefit to treatment. Most women spend a lot on skincare these days, so it would seem sensible to show them which products were particularly suited to help with cancer skin problems.

Vision loss

Valda woke up one morning, and could only see a grey film out of her right eye.

'My oncologist told me he had never seen this before, and didn't think it was caused by tamoxifen, which he had started me on a few days before.

Luckily I knew the Reverend David Brown, ex-Chaplain of the Royal Marsden Hospital. He had been on the Ethical Committee at the Marsden that had approved tamoxifen. Looking up his notes, he told me that this had been a recognized side effect. I went to see a French professor, Michel Guillon, who has a private practice just off London's Sloane Square. He said immediately he knew all about eye problems related to tamoxifen. At the end of my examination, he leaned back in his chair and breathed a sigh of relief. Telling me he had been worried that it might be tamoxifen poisoning, which apparently affects about *one in a million, he said it was only a side effect and would disappear within a couple of months . . . But why didn't my oncologist know of this, if both the Chaplain and the professor knew?'*

Weight gain

Weight gain is one thing just about every cancer patient has in common. This is a common side effect of all the drugs, but as Rosemary says: *'My lovely consultant's reply [to my complaint] was "Do you want to be fat and alive, or thin and dead?"'* Go to Chapter 14 (page 98) for more about food and sensible eating.

Helpful therapies

Hormonal drugs can have very strong and nasty side effects, but using specially-developed therapies – such as massage – not only help with side effects, they help you to stay on these life-extending drugs, and give you a 'feel good' boost.

If you can't get help here with skin problems, and if you can afford the cost and the time, go to France or Germany. Their medical spas are excellent at dealing with skin problems. There's more information about this on page 106.

Sun is an enemy

Outside, even in winter, it makes sense to use a moisturiser with a sun protection factor of at least 15 on your face every day, and a minimum of Factor 30 when in the sun. And use a fake tan if you want to, NEVER a sunbed.

And remember . . .

Cancer Research UK's findings are that side effects show that the drugs are working, so if you are sick, or if break out in skin lesions or have a scalding hot flush, the scientists say you should be happy!

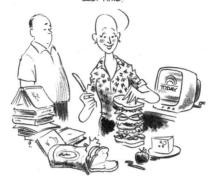

Chapter 10

Complementary Therapies

There is a move to lump complementary and alternative medicine together, and to call it CAM. I'm totally against this. Professor Edzard Ernst, the first Professor of Complementary Medicine in the United Kingdom, says the simplest definitions are:

Complementary is as an adjunct to conventional treatment.
Alternative is a substitute for conventional treatment.

In other words, complementary medicine works with ordinary medicine; alternative medicine is a substitute – and you must be careful when you use it.

When Valda finished her radiotherapy treatment, she felt like a wet rag, so her doctor suggested that she take advantage of complementary therapies on offer at a local private cancer centre.

'I was intrigued. Being British, I had never had massage as part of medical treatment, but found that it was normal in other countries. I then found Cancer Research UK says, "Generally, massage therapy can help lift your mood, improve your sleep and enhance your well being. There is some evidence to help support these benefits."

Then, on holiday in Germany, I found the huge rehabilitation centre Klinic Bad Sulza [see page 109], where they give these therapies as normal treatment. It is partially funded by the German Health Service and partially by German insurance companies – and we all know insurance companies don't pay for anything if it isn't effective. I was introduced to a range of massage therapies, and found they really helped – with fatigue, with sleeping, and with general well-being.

When I returned I was determined to keep up the good work and have a monthly massage. Now I am on Aromasin®, the side effects are still not nice, but I know that if I start getting grumpy and extra tired, it is the end of the month and I am due for a massage.'

Massage

Massage has been used as a therapy for thousands of years. In other European countries, particularly in France or Germany, it is often provided as part of the care package whilst you are on drugs. In some countries you get this on the health service, or it is paid for by insurance!

However, there is a myth going round in some medical circles that cancer patients should not have massage – it might spread the cancer cells.

At an NHS meeting of eminent professors discussing clinical trials, Tim raised the subject of massage – a recognized complementary therapy. '*The Macmillan representative slated me, saying that this was not advised. She wouldn't listen to me when I said that Macmillan had published research into massage which showed how beneficial it was for cancer patients – abroad it can often be provided by health services, and why was I having massage provided and paid for by Macmillan?*'

This attitude is not unusual, so when you start exploring this side of treatment, watch out for:

- Ignorance
- Lack of specific knowledge of massage therapies available
- Lack of understanding of the benefits of each therapy

These myths are gradually being dispelled, but you do need to make sure that your therapist understands cancer – and knows what type of massage to give you.

A good therapist will have studied the needs of cancer patients, or perhaps works at a local hospice or cancer centre, so understands what is required.

Massage treatments in Germany and France

The German Cancer Information Service says:

> 'Patients can obtain massage if it is approved by their doctor, also on a regular basis, and if their health insurance covers it, or if they pay for it themselves. The decision if a patient is entitled to massages is made by the attending physician on the basis of medical necessity. He also determines how many massages for an individual patient are medically necessary, and over what period of time.'

Talking to therapists in Germany, some told me that they often give massages to British patients, and say the only difference is that English men keep their socks on when told to undress!

In France they seem to have the same sensible approach to massage, and looking at their cancer care you can understand why celebrities such as Kylie Minogue and Marianne Faithfull, although living near UK cancer centres, decided to be treated in France.

Every cancer treatment centre I visited in France offered specially tailored massages – and they were excellent. You are often given massage under jets of warm spa water and, surprisingly, this leaves your skin beautifully soft.

How to find appropriate massage in Britain

As a cancer patient, you need to find a therapist who is:

- trained in dealing with the special problems caused by cancer
- able to help with build-up from toxins
- able to help with fatigue
- able to deal with extremely dry skin
- skilled in coping with broken, bruised or bleeding areas
- able to give suitable massage – not deep massage

Cancer Research UK says you should NOT have massage if you:

- are still undergoing cancer treatment
- are very weak
- have bone fractures
- have heart problems
- suffer from arthritis
- are pregnant or breast-feeding.

If you are still having radiotherapy, the treatment area should be avoided.

Lymphoedema

There is a particular type of massage used for this. Make sure your therapist understands the condition and is properly trained, otherwise they could do more harm than good. They will probably use the Vodder method, which is the best known massage for this condition.

If you have lymphoedema, and cannot get treatment on the NHS, go to my web page, www.after-cancer.com/lymphoedema for details of whom to write to. Others have followed this route, and the NHS has paid for private treatment – so, good luck!

What benefits does massage give you?

It is real YOU time, when you are the total and complete focus of the therapist. It is excellent for de-stressing and many patients say that it helps with fatigue. And you feel good afterwards. So, if you are offered massage therapy at a cancer centre or cancer hospital, take it! Often they will give you a certain number of treatments for free, and then you may be able to pay for more. If you are not offered it or choose to go elsewhere, there are good salons all over Britain. Many excellent companies supply trained staff to franchises, such as Decleor, Clarins, Aveda, and Elemis. Just ensure that the therapist has had proper training. They should:

- ask you to fill out a questionnaire
- insist on a letter from your medical team
- take time to find out your requirements.

If you are visiting London, I highly recommend you take a trip to the Elemis Day Spa, just off Bond Street (0870 410 4210), where they offer the Rolls-Royce of treatments. Elemis also make products that help with extra dry skin, and I love their face mask and body scrub, which get rid of scaly skin patches. www.elemis.com 01278 727830.

If you have a beauty training school near you with a good reputation, they may offer free aromatherapy massage. The downside is that you are treated in a class laid out like a slab of meat with others in rows, but it is free (although a small tip is accepted gratefully by the student). Before you go, do check out the school's credentials with the local authority that regulates the school, and also ask your oncology specialist.

For more information, or to find a practitioner contact the General Council for Massage Therapy, www.gcmt.org.uk, 0151 430 8199.

Facial massage

Some people think a facial is pure indulgence. My feeling is that sensible patients realize that it is vitally important to look after your facial skin. It is exposed to the elements on a daily basis, and if you get cracked skin or it wrinkles up, it gives an open invitation to encourage infection and other problems. Hormonal drugs generally dry out facial skin, giving you so-called 'brillo pad' skin, so it needs feeding from the inside *and* the outside.

Feeding from within is basically drinking plenty of pure water, and eating sensibly. Feeding from outside involves having a good skincare routine and using good skincare products.

However much you try to feed and look after your skin, you really should find the time and funds for a monthly facial. Do this, and you will not only feel better, you'll look better!

Aromatherapy massage

This is when the therapist uses a combination of sweet-smelling plant oils. Patients talk of short-term 'de-stressing' effects from the smell, and the oils certainly enhance the feeling of well-being that comes with a massage.

Reflexology

This is when a therapist uses his or her fingers and thumbs to put pressure on different points on the soles of your feet. Cancer Research UK says that a study in 2007 found that reflexology given by partners reduced pain and anxiety in people with metastatic cancer, but they admit that they need more research to know if it really does help people with cancer.

Personally, it annoys me that I can't find a scientific explanation why this works – but it works for me. Studies are being undertaken in a Glasgow hospital on treating constipation using reflexology, and different people will tell you they have different benefits from this treatment.

Relaxation therapy

This is supposed to help you relax both your body and your mind. If you are a good subject, it could be helpful for a range of problems, especially if you are stressed. Go with an open mind. If it doesn't work – you are not alone.

Art therapy

Professor Michael Baum is an example of how much time and trouble some people take over helping patients on our recovery path. He set up art therapy at the Royal Marsden Hospital and has kindly allowed me to quote an extract from his book, *Breast Beating* (Anshan, ISBN 978 1848290 426)

'Some time in 1990, shortly after I was appointed Professor of Surgery at the Royal Marsden Hospital, I was making a solitary ward round, checking on the welfare of my breast cancer patients, when I came upon an unfamiliar woman handing out pots of paint to a patient recovering from my surgical assault.

Assuming she was an occupational therapist and wanting to make my presence felt, I engaged her in conversation. Within five minutes of talking to Camilla Connell, I was totally won over to the concept of art therapy for patients with cancer. Since that day, a warm relationship has developed between us, based on mutual respect and understanding for the contributions we can each make to patients recovering from cancer surgery, or for that matter, any other life-threatening disorder.

My interest and enthusiasm can be described at two levels. First, there is an uncanny thematic similarity running through the works of many of these patients who face serious disease. It is as if the experience of cancer stimulates some deeply hidden communal memory to evoke the symbolism of life and death, fear and hope. The tree, for example, is a recurring theme in these works of art, one that can be traced back through many cultures to the original 'etz chaim' (tree of life) of the Old Testament.

At an individual level, what I have found so moving is the obvious cathartic value of using art to express hidden fears, the progression of the imagery from fear to hope as a sign of recovery and sadly, in the reverse direction, as a sign of deterioration. There is no doubt that art is a powerful medium for self-expression for frightened patients who do not have the words or the will to express themselves verbally.

Many patients have hidden talents, yet even in the absence of conventional artistic skill some of their almost childlike and naïve pictures are enormously expressive and deeply moving to the observer. I believe that art therapy is a unique vehicle for allowing patients with cancer to express hidden emotions and thus, to some extent, provide their own psychotherapy . . .

Good medicine is not only the practice of the science of the subject, but also the practice of the humanities of the subject. Central to the humanitarian practice of medicine is the development of good communication skills. Central to the development of good communication skills is the development of empathy. Strictly, empathy means trying to get inside the patient's head, to feel his or her fears and pain, a task that even the most empathetic of doctors can find extremely difficult. As far as I am concerned, art therapy is the most direct line into the patient's experience of illness, and I feel almost ashamed that I do not make use of it in the day-to-day practice of my own clinic. Perhaps there simply are not enough Camilla Connells to go round. If there were, I have little doubt that the drugs' budget for the NHS would fall, as prescriptions for anxyolitics and anti-depressants would be replaced by the prescription of art therapy.

You can see an interview with Professor Baum on www.youtube.com. Type into the search box 'Prof.Michael Baum interview, Richard Dawkins' and it should take you there.

To find out more about complementary medicine, you can contact the British Complementary Medical Association, www.bcma.co.uk, 0845 345 5977, or you could also contact the Research Council for Complementary Medicine, www.rccm.org.uk, 020 7833 8897.

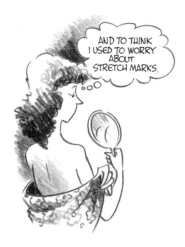

Chapter 11
Alternative therapies

Alternative medicine is generally a term used in the western world to cover any healing practice that does not fall within the realms of conventional medicine. There are literally hundreds of alternative therapies and treatments, ranging from naturopathy, chiropractic, herbalism, traditional Chinese medicine, Unani, Ayurveda, meditation, yoga, biofeedback, hypnosis, homeopathy, acupuncture, and diet-based therapies, in addition to a range of other practices.

What they have in common is that:

- devotees swear by them
- few have been clinically tested.

Breakthrough Breast Cancer does not advocate the use of alternative therapies. However, when the 'production line' that is cancer treatment makes you feel de-humanized, you can turn to anyone who makes you feel better. And this is where alternative therapy practitioners come in. They focus solely on you, and the 'feel good' factor can be wonderful – a great boost.

My e-mail inbox is full of offers of the latest 'cancer' treatment, from goji berries to vitamin supplements. They seem to have worked for the person e-mailing but they are not for me. Most alternative treatments are not proven, and what makes one person feel good, may not work for the next patient. I even get e-mails offering 'life-enhancing' treatments at some exotic resort or hotel. I look at the credentials of the directors to see if any have recognized medical qualifications. Usually they don't, so I delete them straight away. Anyone relaxing in a tropical paradise being pampered by attentive staff should feel good. But life-enhancing? That feeling may only last as long as the flight home.

Many alternative therapies, supplements and pills are offered on the web from sites designed to look folksy and amateurish. They offer 'natural' products, or use other terminology to make it seem that their offering is an alternative to proven therapies and drugs. Be very sceptical – some of the companies could be large corporations making millions.

Associated Press recently published a report on many of these 'natural' products, which quoted Kathy Allen, a dietitian at Moffitt Cancer Center in Florida. She said:

> 'People need to be sceptical of the term "natural". Supplements lack proof of safety or benefit. Asked to take a drug under those terms, most of us would say no. When it says "natural", the perception is there is no harm. And that is just not true.'

The report then gave two website addresses for more information: an anti-scam site, www.quackwatch.com, and tips from US Food and Drug Administration www.cfsan.fda.gov/DMS/ds-savvy.html.

My personal feeling is that if you think something is doing you good, go for it, as long as it does not conflict with your current treatment. So before you buy any supplements, check with your doctor. You must think very hard before you decide to stop conventional treatment and replace this with alternative therapies. Do some real research – and don't believe all that you see on alternative centres' websites. There is often another side to a story.

Also, many alternative therapies cost a lot of money. Is it really worth it, or would you be better off using a complementary therapy, such as massage, to give you the 'feel good' factor?

A question asked on the website Yahoo Answers gives a very good indication of what bothers the unscientific world health-wise:

Question: I'm doing a paper on traditional cancer treatments vs alternative treatments vs no treatment at all. Which is best in your opinion? Where do you find information on things like this?

The person who asked the question chose this as the best answer she received:

Answer:

1. Conventional cancer treatments such as chemotherapy and radiotherapy have been tested and proven in double-blind clinical trials. We know they are not perfect, and have side effects, but they have been tested and proven that they save many lives and prolong many, many more.

2. Alternative treatments are treatments that have never been tested in that way, and have never been proven to be effective against any cancer. If they had been, they wouldn't be 'alternative medicine', they would just be medicine. Alternative, in this context, is just another word for unproven. Sadly, wherever there is cancer there is an unscrupulous charlatan eager to make money from desperate and vulnerable people, selling them ineffective and sometimes dangerous alternative 'cures'.

3. No treatment at all? Barring a miracle – and you know how rare they are – that means certain prolonged and possibly painful death.

Why are medics so sceptical?

They are scientists, and science looks for proof. Approved clinical trials under strictly controlled conditions are one way of proving a medicine or treatment works. But alternative medicine does not provide this.

Why you should be sceptical

As a cancer patient you are very vulnerable. Helena and Ingrid had been through cancer together:

'We were both diagnosed with exactly the same breast cancer, at *the same time. I listened to my oncologist, and finally made up my mind that I would start on tamoxifen, even though I was warned that the side effects might not be nice. But looking at the statistics for the clinical trials, it seemed the more sensible option.*

Ingrid told me I was stupid. She kept on bombarding me with e-mails saying she was trying this and that – and eventually went off to Thailand for some sort of 'light therapy', costing over £20,000.

Just recently she phoned me – her cancer has returned. I felt so sorry for her, but was glad I hadn't followed her path. I don't know if her cancer was due to return anyway, but...'

Trick or Treatment

Anyone considering an alternative therapy should read a book called *Trick or Treatment* written by Dr Simon Singh and Professor Edzard Ernst (Bantam Press, ISBN 978-0-59306-129-9). Professor Ernst was the world's first Professor of Complementary Medicine, and now works at the Peninsula Medical School at Exeter. Their aim with the book is to *'promote analytical thinking, and to be neither promotional nor derogatory but to struggle for objectivity.'* They have spent the past 15 years testing the therapies, treatments and supplements we are offered. The book explains and tests the theory behind alternative medicines, and analyses if they work by evaluating scientific research.

They have come to the conclusion that most of these treatments just don't work. Some of those on which whole cancer treatments are based are discredited, and some are described as 'potentially harmful'. Many so-called cancer centres are not going to like what is written about them, but do read the book – you could save yourself a fortune, if nothing else.

I loved their description of Feng Shui, *'. . . based on biologically implausible concepts and there is no evidence to show that it works. A competent interior designer can probably offer equally good advice . . . no evidence to show it does anything but enrich those who promote it.'*

Colonic irrigation and other treatments, such as coffee enemas, are de-bunked and dismissed. Of colonic irrigation they say it is *'ineffective and dangerous'.*

On fashionable detox treatments, their comment is, *'The only substance that is being removed from a patient is money.'*

Mainstream massage is explained in a simple way, and the book tells you which ones are useful, and which just sound nice but are not proven to be effective.

To conclude

Sometimes medics are their own worst enemies, and their 'couldn't care' attitude pushes patients towards alternative treatment. They don't spend enough time trying to understand our fears and concerns. So patients who are lost and frightened may turn to a nice therapist with the wonderful 'new' idea to help. And it may help. Losing fear and despondency could help them to blossom, certainly if they were going to get better anyway.

So, whilst I don't decry alternative treatments, they should be taken cautiously, and are not for the majority. Belief is a strange but potent force, and what works for someone because they believe in it, should not be lauded as *the* cancer treatment – because as *Trick or Treatment* proves – it so often isn't.

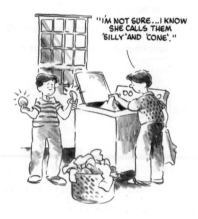

Chapter 12

Using the web

Breast Cancer Care ran an online survey, asking where people looked for information. The survey found:

- 11 per cent get their information from medical professionals
- 13 per cent from publications
- 74 per cent off the web

One would expect a high percentage to say the web but even so the results highlight the fact that many people turn to the internet for information. Some doctors speak disparagingly of the information found on the net, but for many of us, it is a lifeline.

Getting on the web

If you can't work a computer, you will be surprised how many silver surfers learn to do this when faced with cancer. There are plenty of ways to learn – a family member, adult education classes, or from your local library. Some charities might even teach you. Why bother? Because doctors say the better informed you are, the more you can help yourself on your cancer journey. And today, there is a huge amount of excellent and helpful information on the internet.

There are also forums where you can 'chat' to fellow patients, and if you live on your own this is a way of feeling you are not alone.

Buying a computer

Today, the assistants in computer stores have learnt to speak plain English not 'geek speak'. Stores such as PC World are now much more 'user-friendly' and there is a lot of help available. I went into my local branch of PC World the other day and asked the salesman for a laptop. He showed me rows of gleaming machines. Right in the middle was a bright pink Sony Vaio. The thought of opening this up in the business class of Eurostar when all the 'suits' got out their latest black and silver gizmos was irresistible. Without a doubt, that was the one I wanted. The manager came over, totally bemused. Didn't I want to know how many gigabytes it had? No. What extra features it had? No. My theory was that all machinery today goes wrong at some time, so why not have fun in the meantime! And I couldn't have written this book without it.

One other thing. Regardless of what the salesmen tell you, gizmos always go wrong, so I signed up to a fantastic telephone helpline service called 'The Tech Guys' (www.thetechguys.com). These are experts, based in Nottingham, who are brilliant at calming you down. Then they 'take over' your computer by remote control, whilst you sit back and watch as they click backwards and forwards sorting out your problems.

There are many other support services, and if you are new to computers, it is a good idea to sign up to one.

Research on the web

Today, with new cancer drugs coming on-stream constantly, good medicine practice often develops into a patient/doctor partnership, with more informed patients discussing the possibilities of different treatment options with their medical staff.

However, you must beware of following 'airy fairy' theorists and those with a weird axe to grind. There are a lot of charlatans out there with very dubious websites – so question what you read. Try and find out if an official source backs up the information you gather, before you ask your medical team to look at something you have found on the web.

If we use the web sensibly, we can become far better informed as patients, which is to everyone's benefit. If something has rave reviews, dig around to find out who funded the research and who is paying to put this up on the web. When reading testimonials, look for authoritative research that has been carried out to back up claims. You soon realize that many so-called hospitals and centres are only in this for what they can get out of it. You can easily check the name and qualifications of a hospital and doctor – and soon you will develop a sixth-sense to root out suspect 'research'.

Where to start?

The world's major cancer charities and hospitals all have good websites, with well-researched information. All these are listed in the web addresses in Chapter 18. If you are being treated in one country, there is nothing to stop you from trawling the web to access information from another country's official sites. Most will have an English language version – just look for a British or US flag somewhere on the site.

Search for information that will be helpful for you, such as:

1. a new drug that you heard someone mention
2. benefits that can be obtained from a certain treatment
3. handling side effects

Often drugs are clinically trialled, and you can go on the web to find out how these trials are progressing. If you can't find anything, ask your oncologist. Some medical websites may require you to pay for access – but you should be able to do this for free in the hospital. If you can't, ask why.

Be careful – if the website is hosted by the drug company that is developing the drug, they may have a vested interest. Also, beware of websites that:

*   are only there to sell you a theory – usually very off-beat
*   are self-published by someone who wants to promote their ideas, and are not backed up by evidence of clinical trials
*   offer a 'new' or 'miraculous' cure or treatment for cancer
*   promote over-priced goods.

Forums

If you want to chat with fellow cancer sufferers, every major cancer charity has forums. These are very mixed; some are for posting queries to ask others for information about a little-known problem, others are there as an emotional crutch.

Look at the forums carefully. Read what people have posted to decide if the forum is suitable for you. Some postings are badly written ramblings, and can be boring, as people write up their day-to-day diaries. Others post strange and disturbing theories, which could upset you. However, if you persevere, eventually you will find a forum that 'fits' what you want. Those run by the major charities usually have a moderator who oversees what is written.

You can post queries on a forum, for example to ask if anyone is on a certain trial, or whether anyone has any experience of a particular drug.

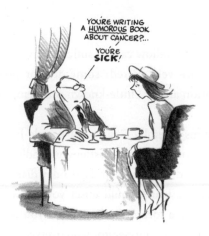

Chapter 13

Friends and family

One of the most common ways of handling cancer is to withdraw into yourself. You have been hit with a massive 'whammy' and you don't want to be a burden to friends and family, so you crawl into a shell and won't let anyone help.

That's not good for you or your friends. They want to help, and they would expect you to do the same for them, so don't be proud – or ungracious. Refusing help because you are embarrassed is stupid, and throws someone's thoughtful gesture back at them – they may have been agonizing for days, trying to think what to do.

It's you with cancer this time – next time it could be your friend. So set out some ground rules that will help you and everyone else.

Making lists

You are going to need help and support, so it can be helpful to give a friend or partner a list of the things you would like help with. That way, when friends ask what they can do, it is easy for them to make suggestions. If you know you are having a course of radiotherapy, you could make plans for friends to pick up the kids from school or buy your weekly groceries.

Advice for friends

If you are a friend, don't just say, 'Let me know if I can help.' Offer to do something in particular, such as, 'Can I walk the dog every day until you finish treatment?' You know your friend's lifestyle. If they enjoy a regular manicure, but won't be able to drive to the salon, offer to drive them – or even to come over to the house and do it yourself. This is just an example, but if you think of what you would want if this happened to you, it is easy to come up with ideas.

Remind them you exist as a friend. For me, the things I really enjoyed were receiving funny cards. I never knew when one would arrive, so hearing the post through the letterbox was a lovely time of anticipation. I was very tired, so just opening a card and sitting down to read a short message was all I could manage – then I would sit and laugh and think.

My friend Thirza was fantastic. Every time she went near a shop that sold figs (one of my favourite treats) she would buy half a dozen, and hang them in a plastic bag on the doorknob as she went past my home. She knew I was often sleeping, so this way I wasn't disturbed, but when I came out of the house there was a lovely present. Another friend loved her garden, and having no energy to tend it upset her more than her treatment – until her friends organized a rota to make sure it looked its best.

To be useful, you may need some basic information. Your friend might be very private and may not want you to know all about their situation. But here are things you may want to consider:

- Who is going to look after your friend during the day?
- Will they be able to prepare their own meals, or will they welcome help?
- Will any children need to be taken to and from school? Will they need help with homework?
- Do they have a partner who is physically fit or are there things that they might need help with?
- Are there changes that need to be made in the home? Is there equipment that could help the person to do things more easily?
- Might they need help getting financial support? (Tact required!)

If your friend does not open up to you, they may discuss difficulties with a professional. It might be possible to talk to doctors or social workers. It's a difficult balance, but if you are a true friend, you will work something out.

Decide what you can and want to do.

- What are you good at?
- Are you handy around the house? Could you put up handrails or wheelchair ramps if needed?
- Could you house-sit, babysit or dog-sit, so their partner can visit them in hospital?
- Could you take the children out for the day to give the parent(s) some time together?
- Would you be prepared to pay for, say, a cleaner for half a day a week to help out?
- Could you get relevant booklets or information for your friend?
- Can you find videos, CDs or DVDs that they like?
- Do they need the furniture rearranged (for instance, so that the patient can sleep on the ground floor because they cannot manage stairs). If so, could you help them to do it?
- Will there be groceries (such as bread and milk) or flowers at home when the person gets out of hospital?
- Even a simple gesture such as offering family members a lift to and from the hospital can be helpful.
- And if you give flowers (a lovely thought) try to ensure they are 'ready tied' so they can be put straight into a vase, or, better still, that are already in water, so your friend just has to place them where they look good. It can be difficult lifting up long flower stems to arrange them in a vase.

Look at the list of the things you are prepared to do, and start by offering one or two of them. Offering all of them at once may overwhelm your friend.

Pick some small tasks that are practical but that your friend might not be able to do for themselves easily. It is important that you actually do whatever you offer to do and don't aim to do too much.

It may need a little thought and some inside knowledge. For example, if your friend likes her hair done every week, it is easy to arrange this in hospital – most hospitals have this service, or can call it in, and it is a nice, thoughtful touch.

If children are involved, they may need to talk to someone. Often a child will open up to a family member or older family friend when they are frightened of asking their parent difficult questions. They are going to feel very upset that a beloved parent is sick and sometimes might even feel it could be their fault. They need support and someone to be there for them when they need to talk. As well as helping with babysitting, school pick-ups and homework, you could also get them to help you cook something for their parent. It is surprising how much fun they will have, especially if they would never think of helping at home! It will also make them feel useful.

Time is a valuable gift. The important thing is to be reliable and there for your friend.

One of the good things that comes from having cancer is that you find out who are your real friends!

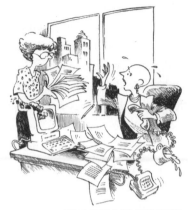

"NOT NOW... I'M HAVING A NO HAIR DAY!"

Chapter 14

Food, glorious food

During treatment you often have to force yourself to eat. Drugs can make you lose your sense of taste and smell, and your appetite disappears. Nurses can tell you what food supplements you can buy to make up the shortfall. Frankly, often you just want to glug down the mixture quickly, knowing you must keep up your strength.

Kind friends may cook lots of delicious meals, but after a mouthful you may not feel like eating more. This happens, so just explain and put the rest into the freezer to heat up another time. Your friend will understand.

Valda had this problem:

> Sadly, the only thing I fancied was chocolate. Now, if drugs had given me an aversion to such fattening food there might have been some point!"

Hormonal drugs have funny side effects. Peppers, chillies, e-numbers and food additives can react strongly and make you sick. Everyone is different, but when you look at your favourite dish and feel you couldn't touch a mouthful, this is often your brain telling you something will react with the drugs.

One patient said that she developed an aversion to whatever she had eaten the day before each chemo treatment. So, if you like food that is good for you, perhaps it is best not to eat it before treatment!

Valda says:

> '*Treatment made me realize what is pumped into our food. I love salmon, but one evening eating some farmed salmon in a smart restaurant sent me rushing for the bathroom. Eventually I found that I could tolerate organic farmed salmon but anything else fed on pellets was a no-no. I also realized that as I wasn't eating much (although the drugs made me put on weight), it was best to make sure that what I ate was the best possible. Organic food often tasted nicer, and insisting on free-range chickens and eggs meant I did my little bit for animal welfare. Eating organic meat made me feel good, but I must admit my taste buds couldn't tell the difference. However, friends starting remarking on how good my roasts tasted – so there is obviously a difference.*'

Dieticians will give you tons of advice, which can sometimes be contradictory. What you need to do is to look sensibly at your diet and try, as much as possible, to eat organically, with meat that is free of hormonal additives.

You will probably find that your appetite has reduced, and big helpings, even of your favourite foods, are left half-eaten. This is your body saying 'enough is enough', and in some way compensates for the weight gain that comes with most drugs.

Vitamins

Cancer patients get a massive amount of advice from friends about vitamins they should take, but current thinking in research centres is that you are unlikely to need extra vitamins, as long as you are eating plenty of fruit and vegetables, and eat a sensible, varied diet. So, unless the doctor advises you to take a certain vitamin, forget expensive supplements and grab a few more grapes.

Lycopene has been feted as a wonder food – a powerful antioxidant found naturally in tomatoes. However, the fruit is better for you, and cheaper.

Mediterranean diet

A study reported in the British Journal of Cancer recommended a Mediterranean diet, saying fruits, vegetables, cereals and fish are good, as is eating less red meat. Another study also commends broccoli.

There is no one 'superfood' that can stop you developing cancer, but if you eat healthily, you have a better chance of a good recovery. The healthier your body is, the more reserves you have to fight nasty 'invasions'.

If you like meat, try things like kidneys and liver. Lambs' kidneys are incredibly cheap, and can be cooked in olive oil. Peas and beans also score highly.

What else to eat

You have probably been bombarded with diet sheets. Friends add to the confusion by telling you about articles they have read, suggesting things you should and should not eat. During my cancer journey, I was given diet sheets and advice from six different hospital dieticians – advice that sometimes contradicted their colleagues. So now I just eat what I want, which basically follows the usual diet eaten around the Mediterranean. Luckily I do love fruit and vegetables!

Milk

Michel Montignac was the French scientist who first took on the Canadian research into low glycaemic index foods, and developed a diet that has kept French women slim for twenty years. I asked him what he was up to now.

'Milk,' he said. He couldn't understand why a food that for centuries had been regarded as essential for life, has suddenly been demonized. So he is carrying out detailed research on milk and dairy produce. Although milk doesn't feature so much in a Mediterranean diet, yoghurt is a staple.

He strongly suspects that the problems being reported as being the fault of dairy produce – allergies etc – are in fact caused by the way that cows are reared today. Many are reared on hormones and antibiotics, kept indoors all year round, and fed on 'made up' foods. He strongly advocates that we don't forsake milk (unless we really have a dairy allergy) but instead change to organic milk.

So far, what I have read about organic milk bears out what he says. In her book *Eat Your Heart Out* (Penguin, 978-0141026015), Felicity Lawrence says that 'You are what you eat' applies to cows as much as humans. In the past 60 years the iron content of milk appears to have dropped by more than 60 per cent. It has lost 2 per cent of calcium and 21 per cent of its magnesium. On the plus side, if you drink organic milk, a recent study showed that on average, a pint of organic milk contained 68 per cent more omega-3 fatty acids than conventional milk.

Fruit and vegetables

We all know they are good for us and now there are companies who will provide boxes of organic produce delivered to your door on a regular basis. This is such a sensible idea. Once a week – or daily if you wish – a box of lovely, seasonal and, where possible, locally sourced fruit and vegetables arrives on your doorstep. No lugging home heavy apples and pears. Order extra bananas, because nutritionists tell you they are excellent food if you are too tired to eat.

If you have too much, get out the organic milk and make a milk shake. Pour a glass of milk into the blender, add any excess fruit, and for more energy, add a teaspoon of honey. Whizz up and enjoy!

However, beware the press releases extolling the virtues of fruit as an anti-cancer cure. So far, none of the reputable research institutes offer any evidence that this is so. What they do say is that the more fruit and vegetables you eat the better your health and therefore the better chance you have of recovery.

Peppers, chillies or garlic

You may find that hormonal drugs disagree violently with chillies, garlic or peppers. All three can be found in many sauces, and in ready-meals and restaurant dishes, so check before you throw up! Most restaurants are used to the British dislike of garlic, so won't mind if you ask them to go easy on this if it makes you sick.

If you cook, substitute garlic, peppers and chillies with herbs, rocket, watercress and other 'peppery' salad vegetables.

Grapefruit

An undoubtedly healthy fruit but it can react with certain drugs, so make sure that yours are safe before eating it.

Meat

Recently I had a seven-hour heart operation. Afterwards, there was the usual packet of pills. When I complained that 20 different ones were too many, my surgeon looked at me quizzically. 'Do you eat meat?' he asked. Yes! So he advised me to eat liver, kidneys and a limited but regular amount of lean meat. This was to restore whatever minerals were lacking – and I could throw away half the pills.

So I asked Alison Jee, meat expert, for her advice:

> *'For everyone, the quality of the meat they eat is paramount. If you have or are recovering from cancer it is even more important to choose top quality produce. Choose a butcher like Broad Stripe Butchers www.broadstripebutchers.co.uk.'*

Broad Stripe Butchers are an on-line British butchers. They realized that more people were looking for the kind of wonderful quality and lovingly selected meat that top chefs, such as Gordon Ramsay, were choosing.

Calcium-rich foods

Osteoporosis is a bone-thinning disease we are told we *might* get as a result of taking hormonal drugs. You can't avoid it, if it is going to happen, but the National Osteoporosis Society recommends a healthy, balanced, calcium-rich diet combined with lots of weight-bearing exercise, like walking.

Adults should aim to eat 700mg of calcium every day. You can find calcium in a wide range of foods such as:

- milk and dairy products, especially the low-fat varieties
- green leafy vegetables (watercress, okra, spinach)
- dried fruit (dried figs, apricots and currants – five figs provide 250mg of calcium)
- tinned fish like salmon, sardines, pilchards (provided you eat the bones)
- fried whitebait, sesame seeds and tahini are also high in calcium.

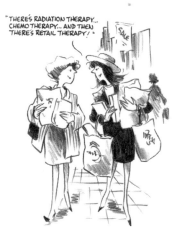

"THERE'S RADIATION THERAPY... CHEMO THERAPY... AND THEN THERE'S RETAIL THERAPY!"

Chapter 15

Taking a break

When you finish hospital treatment, one thing every consultant, doctor and nurse will say is, 'Take a holiday'. But they don't answer the questions that come to mind:

- Can I fly?
- How far should I travel?
- Where should I go?
- Will I get tired?
- How do I get insurance?
- Can I go out in the sun?
- What happens if I get ill again while I'm away?

Can I fly?

Yes, but doctors question the benefit of flying halfway round the world for a holiday, with all the stress that comes with it (not to mention the carbon emissions), only to end up exhausted from jet lag. So keep your travelling time to a manageable length, and consider going by train. By train, you don't suffer from jet lag and you are breathing 'proper' air, rather than very adulterated air that is not good for your health.

How far should I travel?

Doctors who specialize in aviation medicine give the guideline that you need approximately one day to recover from jet lag for every hour flown. By train you get fatigue, but this can be restored with a good night's sleep. Now, thanks to Eurostar (www.eurostar.com), train travel in Europe has had a revival. Rail companies are realizing that it pays to work together to offer travellers seamless travel and make it easier to book and travel by train. European Rail is an excellent company that can tailor-make a train-and-hotel package for you (www.raileurope.com).

One tip when taking Eurostar; ask to change at Lille, if you have to change, rather than Paris. You'll only have a short wait and perhaps a change of platform, rather than a tedious journey across Paris between stations.

Where should I go?

Staying within Europe is the best option, although North Africa and the Canary Islands are only a short flight away.

One of the best solutions is to go off for a break at a medical spa. That way, if something happens, there are doctors on site. European medical spas are nothing like the British version. They are serious, run by doctors, but dedicated to making you feel well and relaxed. In Britain, pampering spas often are given a 'medi' title, but they are not the same. Make sure that if you want and need genuine spa treatments tailored for cancer patients, ask before you book – or you could end up in a British spa that has a tarot card expert as part of their medical team! There is more about medical spas on page 106.

If the effort of going abroad feels too much, stay in Britain. We do live in a beautiful country and there will be no hassles with travel plans, getting jabs, worrying about visas etc.

Will I get tired?

After cancer treatment, it is likely that you will get tired, so take it easy. If you are travelling by train, take a gentle stroll every so often, eat a meal or go to the buffet car for a drink and a sandwich. Doing this helps the journey along and counters fatigue. And, of course, if you want to sleep, the train seat is roomier and more comfortable than a narrow plane seat.

How do I get travel insurance?

NEVER GO ABROAD WITHOUT IT! If you are British, you MUST get a European Health Insurance card (EHIC) to cover you if you need emergency treatment whilst away. This only gives you limited cover, so you need to take out extra insurance to give you full cover and pay for repatriation if you need it. If you do not have an EHIC, your insurance company may bill you if you have treatment that would have been covered by the card. You can apply online at www.ehic.co.uk, or call 0845 606 2030. You can also get an application form from the Post Office.

Trying to find insurance for a holiday can be a nightmare for cancer patients. Cancer charities have been concerned that many post-cancer patients find they are quoted a massive premium, sometimes more than the trip will cost. Others have been refused insurance 'because they didn't tick the right boxes' when interrogated by insensitive call-centre staff. It can be tempting to buy regular insurance without fully declaring your medical history or to rely on your EHIC to cover you if you need treatment. Don't. You could end up with a huge bill!

Now a company called InsureCancer has filled that gap in the market. It offers comprehensive insurance for cancer patients, with each case being individually assessed. The main requirement is that you should be clinically well for your trip (the company may contact your oncologist for information). It has won a Queen's Award for Enterprise for its innovative and excellent service. Not only that, but the premiums reflect the standards of hospital care in your chosen destination, so if the premium is high it is probably because it will cost a lot of money to fly you to a reputable hospital. So it might pay to rethink your destination! Contact them at www.insurecancer.com or on 012252 780190.

Can I go out in the sun?

Check with your doctor, but the answer almost certainly is yes. Warmth and heat are good for you, but be very cautious in sunlight. The sun's rays can reflect off shiny surfaces such as the sea or even concrete – you can be sitting under an umbrella and still get sunburn. Whenever you go out, wear a high factor sun cream (30+) and renew it frequently.

What happens if I get ill again while I'm away?

This probably won't happen, but after treatment the slightest sneeze can have you worrying about your health. This is normal; your body is at a low and your immune system is shot to pieces. So relax and try to push worries to the back of your mind. If you are enjoying yourself, you'll soon forget about that sniffle!

In the unlikely event that you do get ill, that is where your travel and medical insurance comes in.

Medical spas
FRANCE

France has some of the best cancer treatment in the world, and some brilliant medical spas. They realize that if you are on hormonal drugs, the side effects are going to be with you for a long time, and they are working constantly to improve patients' lives. So when you need treatment and help dealing with side effects – or a large dose of TLC – there is nothing to stop you tapping in to their post-cancer treatments.

The best thing to do is to get a letter of introduction from any of your doctors, listing what treatments you have had and send a copy to the Medical Director of your chosen spa. If your doctor considers this nonsense and won't cooperate, then make an appointment to see an English-speaking doctor when you get to the spa and take it from there. You will have to pay a small amount for the appointment, but nothing like what a private doctor's visit costs in the UK.

Once the doctor has assessed you, he or she will assign therapists and other staff to look after you. Many of these speak excellent English, and if not, medicine is international; they know their job, so just leave them to sort out your problems. It helps to take a dictionary or phrase book with you, so you can communicate a little. It is surprisingly easy!

Most of the French medical spas have the word 'Bain' (meaning 'bath') in their names. This is because of the healing thermal waters that were found there. So here are some of my favourites.

Aix-les-Bains (www.aixlesbains.com/english or www.thermaix.com/fr)

The staff at the marvellous spa here are very experienced in treating post-cancer patients, and make a speciality of care for patients with mouth cancers. Their specially developed little machines, that look like dentists' drills, direct streams of warm, healing water directly at the cancer site. You see patients having treatment with smiles on their faces. Their massages are excellent, and give you back your bounce.

This beautiful lakeside spa town has lots to do for the whole family, including cruises on the lake where you may see beavers and other wildlife. There are plenty of places to stay and many people speak English.

Brides-les-Bains (www.brides-les-bains.com/uk/index.php)

This spa town in the Alps is easily reached via any Eurostar or Rail Europe service. The lovely old thermal spa has been sympathetically modernized. Instead of visitors walking sedately around the gardens, today they go skiing in the winter, and indulge in the spa in summer.

The spa is dedicated to helping you lose weight. When you are handed a menu, what looks like incredibly high menu prices are actually calorie counts! You eat dreamy food that does you good! Then you can go back for fantastic treatments that make you feel wonderful, but help the body get rid of toxins from drugs.

For additional luxury, you could stay at the Grand Hotel des Termes. It is one of those grand hotels that has been totally renovated. Slightly less expensive is the Hotel Golf. The bedrooms – especially on the first floor – are huge, and the bath goodies are sumptuous. For self-catering, the British chalet specialists, Lagrange (www.lagrange-holidays.co.uk) have a residence in the centre of the town that has been refurbished to a high standard, yet remains affordable.

La Roche Posay (www.larocheposay.com)

This is one of the best medical spas I have ever visited. After my skin had broken out in lesions all over my body, and my doctor at the Royal Marsden asked me if I wanted to come off my drugs, a friend told me to go to La Roche Posay. The doctors there examined my rough, peeling and horrid skin, took swabs, examined me thoroughly, then sent me off for lovely spa therapies. Nurses asked questions, examined my skin again, checked a massive prescription form the head doctor had written out, then gave me a bag full of La Roche Posay products specially developed to help cancer skin.

I was sharing the experience with French women who had been sent by their doctors to alleviate side effects from their cancer drugs. The only difference between us was that I had to pay. Over 8,000 French people a year will probably get this treatment as part of their health service.

The spa lies in the Poitou-Charente (north-west France), so is less expensive than the spas in the fashionable eastern side, but there is still lots for the family to do. Legend has it that in the Middle Ages, Bertrand du Guesclin stopped to drink the thermal waters when riding through. His horse, suffering from eczema, immersed itself in the water, and was cured. So if the waters are good enough for horses it must be good enough for us!

In 1617, the doctor to Kings Henry IV and Louis XIII analysed the water and was so impressed that the newly-founded Science Academy sent people to test it too, and the spa of La Roche Posay was founded.

They treat all sorts of skin conditions, but I had come to try the treatments using the soothing Selenium-rich water (probably what cured the horse). Fine-jets of the water spray your body as you are being massaged, leaving your skin incredibly smooth. Dermatological wraps and massages are also designed to give you soft skin, and, as they say, 'improve our daily lives'.

La Roche Posay is also the name of an excellent skincare company, started in the town. The products are only sold via chemists, and there are various ranges tailored to specific skin problems. If your skin is extra-sensitive, they even have a special range – Toleriane. You can now get all of these in Britain and, rumour has it, some patients in the UK have been sent to the spa on the NHS for treatment of skin problems. Like all such rumours, the NHS doesn't want this advertised, but it is worth trying at least!

There are many hotels in the town, all within a short walk of the thermal treatment centre.

For more information on French spas, you can try their website, www.france-thermale.org. It is currently only in French but they have a map on which you can click to find out where spas are situated. You can then contact the local tourist centre or request further information in English. Bon voyage!

GERMANY

Klinic Bad Sulza, near Leipzig (www.medicalspa-kbs.com or www.toskanaworld.net/web/en/klinikzentrum/ausstattung.asp)

This clinic is forging links with British cancer treatment centres, and even had lectures from a specialist British therapist on the differences in treating British patients. The main difference, therapists learned with great hilarity, is that Germans are so used to massages that they take off clothes automatically; the British have to be persuaded even to take their socks off! But these therapists have seen it all before, and you soon relax under their skilful and professional care. The Director, Dr Toerpe, is a sports doctor who was in charge of an Olympic team. What he doesn't know about rehabilitation isn't worth worrying about.

I couldn't believe the size of it. The massive 500-bed complex is built around a huge dome, housing five thermal swimming pools. They are filled with thermal waters at 36 degrees, and you could spend all day in them.

In winter, it is great fun to swim outdoors with snow falling, keeping blissfully warm in the water.

If you go there for treatment, your doctor will send your notes, which will have been read thoroughly by your English-speaking doctor, who then devises a schedule giving you two treatment sessions a day. These include different types of massage, special baths – the mud bath is incredibly soothing and fantastic for your skin – and other therapies which you can take if you wish. The basic cost is £99 per person a day, including single ensuite, three meals a day, doctor's supervision and all recommended treatments.

You could pay around £10 a day extra to stay in Haus 2, which is not so clinical and has larger rooms, and then walk in to the village for the evening meal, as the local food served in the Klinic is hearty, to say the least! In the village, there is a castle, with a good restaurant and fascinating little carriage museum, and a gastro-pub called The Old Schoolhouse.

The most expensive building in the complex is the spa hotel, which includes the beauty spa, offering excellent treatments specially aimed at post-cancer patients: manicures, facials (with fantastic results) and other treatments to induce moisture into dry skins.

If you have lymphoedema they are specialists in treating this, but you need to book a stay for at least 18 days.

All treatments can be taken by others in the family, and kids can enjoy the special Kindergarten, as well as take advantage of the massive thermal water pools. Just don't ask German fellow guests how much they are paying: most are getting their stay free on the German health service.

Air Berlin and Ryanair fly near there (Air Berlin definitely wins hands over with their excellent treatment of anyone with the slightest disability), but you can take a train to Weimar near Bad Sulza. Then I suggest hiring a car, as there is so much to see round about.

ITALY

Sardinia has several well-managed Thalassotherapy treatment centres on the coast. These treatments are based on minerals found in seawater.

I stayed at the Hotel Capo d'Orso (you need a car if you stay here) where their Thalassotherapy centre became my haven from the world. You can book through tour operator Just Sardinia (www.justsardinia.co.uk).

SWITZERLAND

Clinique La Prairie (www.laprairie.ch)

If ever I win the lottery I will head straight for Clinique La Prairie, just outside Geneva. Haunt of stars, international politicians and anyone with several thousand pounds to spend on getting into tip-top health, this is where they go for the most fantastic treatments. However, this is probably the most discreet place you will ever find.

The food is low calorie and delicious (they sell an inexpensive but excellent English-language cookbook), the treatments soothe away all aches and pains, and quietly they do a tremendous amount of good for underprivileged children, paid for by the film stars having plastic surgery.

Reckon to pay upwards of £10,000 a week – but after three days there (as their guest, I hasten to add) you'll feel and look fantastic.

Every spa mentioned has marvellous sport and recreation facilities, so you won't see your family as they take off paragliding, canoeing, swimming in fantastic pools, or they could just enjoy the sun, sitting in a café. And you are doing your long-term health a favour by tapping in to the Continental health system.

BRITAIN

*Titanic Spa, Yorkshire (*www.titanicspa.com)
There are many good spas around the country, but I can personally vouch for this one. It is a wonderful little spa at Linthwaite, near Huddersfield. It is tremendously eco-friendly, bringing water up from a bore-hole, using salt-regulated water in the pool (and no chlorine), and they offer the Elemis and Decleor treatments that are proven to do so much good to cancer skins. The therapists are excellent, having all undergone intensive training, and the treatments are not only a treat but also very good for you and your body.

The pool is enormous, with a pool-side lift and underwater music. There are Aqua Aerobics classes held here, which is one of the gentlest but most effective exercise regimes you can take.

HOTELS FOR THE DISABLED

If you have difficulty getting around, here are some British hotels that are fully-equipped to help.

- Leonard Cheshire Park House Hotel, Sandringham, Norfolk. www.parkhousehotel.org.uk, 01485 543 000
- St. Anne's Hotel, St. Anne's-on-Sea, Lancashire. www.st-annes-hotel.com, 01253 713 108
- Leonard Cheshire Cottage, Kirkcudbright, Dumfries and Galloway. www.scot.leonard-cheshire.org.uk, 01387 711 337

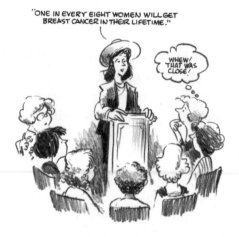

Chapter 16

Paperwork and financial help

Nobody would ever believe the amount of paperwork you will collect on your cancer journey. You will be given so many leaflets, but sometimes they contain useful information. Mark out anything you need to know or may be useful and throw the rest away. Put those you keep in a folder or file. If you just leave them hanging around, sure as eggs is eggs, the one sheet that could be really helpful will have been lost.

If you have a caring partner or friend, you could give them this task. It will give them something concrete they can do to help you and they will remember the information when it is appropriate.

Don't get frustrated by the paperwork. It is improving – gradually. Once, the leaflets were written by doctors. You got a headache trying to understand what they were talking about, and they told you what they thought you should know – not what you wanted to know.

Today, after numerous protests, charities such as Macmillan and Breast Cancer Care are involving patients in writing the copy for information leaflets. And, surprise, surprise, they are more informative. Even doctors read them!

And next time you have some spare minutes in between appointments at the hospital, find out where the information centre is and go and browse through what is available. Many charities put out extremely informative and helpful literature, so dig around to find it.

Help with expenses

Someone said about cancer, '*When you are diagnosed, you enter a whole new world.*' You were probably secure in your family, your home, and most of all with a job that brought in a regular income. Suddenly, you are faced with extra expenses – and, worst of all, you may lose your job. At best your income is reduced, partly because you have to pay out for so many more 'extras', but mostly because you are generally too tired to carry on with a full-time job – at least at the beginning of your treatment.

This is when the various cancer charities can be immensely helpful. Don't feel you can't approach them until you are desperate. It is far more sensible to approach them at the beginning, before any problems start to kick in. You will find that they know all about what is worrying you, and what is more, they often can advise you to do something to avert a possible problem before it becomes overwhelming. They are excellent at giving hints and tips, and suggesting ways to off-set costs. They have lots of ideas to save money that you might never have thought of. What they can do is:

- Give sensible, helpful advice
- Tell you how to get your paperwork in order and help you to fill in forms, if you need it
- Often they have copies of paperwork, which saves you having to run around to obtain this
- Advise on sick pay and benefits, including employment-related benefits, disability and attendance benefits, income support, or tax credits
- Help with NHS costs (car parking, etc)
- Inform you of any grants you may be entitled to
- Give you advice on mortgages, pensions and life assurance
- Give you information on viatical settlements (selling life insurance policies) and how charities can help
- Advise on dealing with debt

Benefits

Here is a basic guide, written by Annie Redmile, who is a whiz at understanding the benefits system.

It is said that money can't buy us everything – but it can help tremendously if you have just been diagnosed with a long-term illness. It may have never occurred to you that you might need special help from others one day, but it can be a very real comfort to learn that money, advice and support is easily accessible.

Of course, there is one inevitability – forms, forms and yet more forms! But there are people to help, and some forms look worse than they really are. With help, it certainly need not be as daunting as you might expect or fear.

Even official government websites can provide helpful information – and there are people and organizations (official and independent) that can help and support you directly.

Most hospitals, and certainly the major ones in big cities, have welfare rights' advisors based on their premises. They also ensure that you are given help and support when you are discharged. The in-house teams are incredibly knowledgeable, understand the system, and have access to the medical staff to obtain supporting letters.

Disability Living Allowance

Disability Living Allowance comes in two parts:
- a mobility component – to help with getting around
- a component to assist with personal care.

Carers' Allowance

There is also a Carers' Allowance, if you have or need a designated carer. If your claim is successful – and there is no reason why it shouldn't be for anyone with a genuinely serious and long-term illness – there may also be an extra amount called a 'severe disability premium' (SDP).

Other Benefits

As you are unlikely to be working when you are ill, there are other possible benefits such as Income Support, Pension Credit, Housing Benefit and Council Tax Benefit. Of course it really can be incredibly stressful battling with all the forms and bureaucracy yourself. Finding the right expert to help and support you is really essential.

Getting help

Citizens Advice Bureau

The Citizens Advice Bureau (CAB) is one of the best-known independent sources of help. There is a national network of over 700 main bureaux and over 1,000 linked outlets giving free advice throughout the UK. It provides free, confidential and impartial advice on virtually any subject – but the main categories of work tend to be in the areas of welfare rights, debt, employment, housing and immigration.

You can find your local CAB through the main national website www.citizensadvice.org.uk or the Scottish site www.cas.org.uk, or you can find the nearest office through a telephone enquiry service. It is important to establish whether you need to make an appointment or whether you can just drop in. Confirming the actual opening times of individual offices is also important.

Websites

There are official government sites about benefits and services, as well as those managed by independent organizations. For example, the official government site, www.direct.gov.uk, is helpful, as is www.benefitsandwork.co.uk. 'Benefits and Work' is an independent site that also has free guides and a membership scheme – £18.55 a year enables its members to receive all printed guides, information obtained through Freedom of Information Act about government departments, access to other members' stories and a members' forum.

Another great site that provides information across the whole spectrum of benefits and grants is www.turn2us.org.uk. It includes a benefits checker, a grants search, and other information and interactive tools covering a wide range of subjects on welfare, benefits, grants and managing money. It is a free service and is all in one place. It is based on highly credible sources and is confidential and secure.

Charities

There are many charities that set out to help people with health problems or those who have to retire early and are finding their finances strained. There are also those who can provide funds for health-specific equipment, such as nebulisers, TENs machines, mobile hoists and electric beds. Guidestar UK, www.guidestar.org.uk, is a website, set up in 2003, dedicated to providing information on every charity and voluntary organization in England and Wales. It publishes easily accessible detailed information about the charities and voluntary sector in the UK.

The Association of Charity Officers, www.aco.uk.net, is a charity that helps other charities, and is a very useful source of information. When you contact them, a member of the ACO will take down a detailed history from you – background, needs, health challenges, etc – and the organization then sets out to research and recommend those charities where you fit with their criteria and who they believe might respond to your needs. You can contact them via e-mail: info@aco.uk.net or by phone 01707 651777

Other available help

Macmillan has a large and very experienced benefits team, especially when it comes to help with the cost of prescriptions, childcare or travel to hospital. They also help with advice on how to cope at work whilst dealing with cancer.

Other ways Macmillan say they can help:

- Find out what benefits are available to you via a guide to the UK benefits system, including help for people of working age, pensioners and carers.
- See what support is available if you are working through cancer, and get further information on the new Employment Support Allowance.
- Talk to other people affected by cancer about the practical issues surrounding cancer in our online communities.
- If you're affected by cancer, a Macmillan benefits adviser can offer specialist advice, available in most areas, on how to ease your financial worries. For general advice on benefits and

financial help, debt and consumer issues, search our financial advice services directory, provided by UK Advice Finder.

- Our benefits awareness e-learning resource is for those who work with people affected by cancer, and aims to raise awareness of the impact that cancer can have on the lifestyles of those affected by cancer, and of the benefits and financial help available to them. You can access this e-learning resource via our Learn Zone.

Macmillan have a guide called 'Help with the cost of cancer'. This is a guide to benefits and financial help for people affected by cancer. You can order a copy from www.macmillan.org.uk, or call 0800 500 800.

Travel and car parks

It can come as an awful shock when you are told you have to go to hospital every day for treatment and you add up what the hospital car park is going to cost! Macmillan are working on this, and thanks to them some hospitals will now waive charges. Do ask.

If you live in London, you can get the Congestion Charges refunded, or the Government may pay, if you are in receipt of benefits. Ask Macmillan or the Cancer Resource Centre for help with claiming this, or there may be a local scheme that covers you. Phone them on 0800 500 800. They are nice helpful people!

If you have to pay ferry or bridge toll charges, again ask your PALS office or the Macmillan Nurse if there are any concessions.

Taxi cards

Some local authorities have an allowance to supply bona-fide taxi journeys for disabled or partly disabled residents. Call to see if you qualify.

And remember, you are not alone. If you find you are having to fight for what is lawfully your right: organizations are there to help. Adela says, *'When I needed the council to do something, their response was, "If we do this for you, it could set a precedent for other disabled people."'* So she phoned Macmillan who offered her a grant. She didn't take it but she used the offer to shame the council into doing what they should be doing. So phone or contact these organizations. They are incredibly helpful.

More helpful contacts in the UK
- Age Concern: www.ageconcern.org.uk, 0800 00 99 66
- Disability Now, magazine and website: www.disabilitynow.org.uk, 020 7619 7323
- Disability Information Services: www.Direct.gov.uk/Disability, 01372 841 395
- RADAR, the disability network: www.radar.org.uk, 020 7250 3222
- Community Legal Service: www.clsdirect.org.uk, 0845 345 4345
- Scottish Legal Aid Board: www.slab.org.uk, 0845 122 8686
- Northern Ireland Legal Services Commission: www.nilsc.org.uk, 028 9040 8888
- Department of Work and Pensions – Disabled People and Carers: www.dwp.gov.uk, 0800 88 22 00. Northern Ireland 0800 22 06 74
- Disability Living Allowance/Attendance Allowance: 08457 123 456
- Carer's Allowance 01253 856 123
- Disability Alliance: www.disabilityalliance.org, 020 7247 8776
- Disability Law Service: www.dls.org.uk, 020 7791 9800
- European Disability Forum: www.edf-feph.org

Pastoral care
Often, your local church or chapel can give help, so it is worthwhile asking. Priests and chaplains are dealing with this type of query all the time.

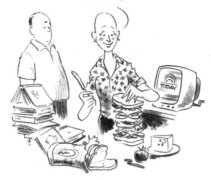

Chapter 17

Regaining your life after treatment

Suddenly you feel you have been let out of school. No more daily trips to the radiotherapy suite. 'Your' chemo chair will be cradling another. The nurses who smiled and joked with you will be smiling at someone else. Your doctor says, *'See you in three months'*. And that's that.

Now you can think of the future, and getting back your life. But, as your doctor may have told you, once you have had breast cancer, you have a higher risk of developing a new breast cancer than someone who has never had the disease – although my oncologist stressed that as I had been on hormonal drugs, these had probably zapped any nasties floating around! However, it is important to continue with the follow-up treatment and care your doctor recommends.

This is also a good time to think about what you are going to do for the future.

Aftercare

Talk to your doctor about follow-ups. Once you leave the hospital cocoon, all sorts of worries surface. Probably the biggest one is, 'Will cancer return?'

No one will promise it won't – but find out from your doctor what to look out for, and if you have regular check-ups, you can ask questions and be reassured.

Very occasionally, breast cancer can come back in the breast or other areas of the body. The symptoms of a cancer recurrence include a new lump in the breast, under the arm, or along the chest wall; bone pain or fractures; headaches or seizures; chronic coughing or trouble breathing; extreme fatigue; and/or feeling ill.

Contact your doctor or breast care nurse immediately if you are worried. Worrying about a recurrence is very common among survivors. My feeling is that medics should learn that there is no use in offering us 'counselling' whilst undergoing treatment, if we don't need it. What we need far more is reassurance after we return home.

Follow-ups

The National Comprehensive Cancer Network has established the following guidelines for follow-up of breast cancer treatment:

1. Have a physical examination performed by a doctor every four to six months for five years.

2. Perform breast self-exam (BSE) every month. For step-by-step breast self-exam instructions, go on the web.

3. Have a mammogram every 12 months. For women treated with breast conserving surgery and radiation therapy, have a mammogram six months after radiation therapy ends, then mammograms of both breasts every 12 months. If you are over 65 in UK, insist that you need this – studies in Sweden and the US say that you should have these yearly until at least 75.

4. Understand which symptoms should be reported immediately:

• Any changes in the remaining breast(s) and chest area, unusual pain, loss of appetite or weight, changes in menstrual periods, unusual vaginal bleeding or blurred vision.

• Dizziness, persistent cough, hoarseness, shortness of breath, headaches, backaches or digestive problems that are unusual or persistent.

5. Have a pelvic exam every 12 months if taking tamoxifen and

have not had the uterus removed. Tamoxifen can increase the risk of uterine cancer, so if you notice anything abnormal, such as vaginal bleeding, tell your doctor or nurse.

6. You are at higher risk of osteoporosis if you are:
   • over 65
   • aged 60-64 with family history or low body weight
   • on aromatase inhibitors, such as anastrozole, exemestane, or letrozole
   • going through treatment-related menopause

   You should have a bone mineral density test every year. Even if you are low risk, you need an office visit to assess osteoporosis risk every year.

Lymphoedema

If lymph nodes were removed as part of the surgery or affected during treatment, lymphoedema (swelling of the hand or arm) may occur. If this happens, contact your doctor IMMEDIATELY, and insist on treatment.

As lymphoedema usually happens long after you have left hospital, it is often difficult to get professional and knowledgeable help. You wander around with a limb so swollen you want to get out a knife to stab it and release the fluid building up so painfully. I managed to get the NHS to pay for private massage treatment by a Vodder-trained physiotherapist. It was well worth the effort and now my legs are almost back to normal.

In the UK, lymphoedema treatment is patchy, and it depends on your Primary Care Trust as to whether they allocate funds for treatment or not. So fight for it, and good luck!

After-effects of radiotherapy

Some weeks or months after you finish radiotherapy, you might experience breathlessness, a dry cough, and/or chest pain. Radiotherapy can cause swelling and fibrosis (hardening or thickening) of the lungs, but symptoms are usually temporary. However, tell your doctor.

Back to work

If you work full time, schedule an appointment with your boss or the human resources department to talk through how you are coping. If you haven't returned to work, discuss when you can do so. Perhaps you could discuss flexitime or part-time until you get stronger, because you are going to be tired both emotionally and physically.

There are horror stories of bosses being totally unsympathetic, probably because of ignorance of cancer. If you are unlucky enough to run up against such a situation, get one of the cancer charities on your side. Most have excellent information on employment rights, and helpful advice about returning to work. If you are being 'frozen out' from your old job, make an urgent appointment with your local Citizens Advice Bureau. It can be time-consuming at first, but they have a wealth of knowledge and can help.

Fatigue

None of the medics told me anything about being tired. But this is something most survivors say 'comes and goes'.

Massage is a wonderful way of coping with fatigue but your body also needs rest. It is old-fashioned, but previous generations knew a thing or two when they went off for naps.

Support groups

There is evidence that people who have support, whether through networking, supportive friends, support groups etc., cope better psychologically with cancer. Some researchers think they may even experience better disease outcomes and live longer, though this is still under study.

If you haven't already done so, investigate joining a support group. There are lots mentioned under Contacts on my website www.after-cancer.com, or ask at your hospital. Don't think it is all counselling and coffee mornings. Most support groups have informed and interesting talks about suitable subjects from a variety of speakers; they often give you massage, organize *Look Good, Feel Better* sessions, and aren't 'do-gooders' at all.

Look Good, Feel Better (www.lookgoodfeelbetter.co.uk) is an international programme that is now in 20 countries, helping women, teens, and even men feel better about themselves while having to deal with the strain of going through chemotherapy or radiotherapy. The programme offers skincare advice, make-up tips and techniques, and help with hair styling. At the end of each session, participants are given make-up kits that would cost over £200 if they bought these for themselves. The kits are made of donations from the multitude of cosmetic companies around the world and many feature in my 'Hero products' in chapter 19.

However, there are people who say support groups aren't useful. In her book *The Secret History of a Woman Patient*, Janet Rhys Dent says her friends told her, she would get 'stuck'. She should get on with real life and forget about her illness. But you can't forget. In fact, you need to be in control to sort out the many little problems that cancer throws up. A good support group can produce informed help, lovely chats, and each time you go there, you usually find someone says something you pick up on.

You might need to try out different groups before settling on one you feel comfortable with. The first one I went to frightened me. Everyone was into exploring their inner soul, and I couldn't understand what they were talking about! Then I joined the Paul D'Auria Support Centre in London (www.pauldauriacentre.org.uk). I liked it so much I am now a Trustee.

Going into the centre, you immediately feel a sense of light and calm. There is a reception area with sofas to flop on, tea and coffee on tap, and a volunteer who smiles and offers help. Here you can sign up for lovely therapies, such as fantastic massages – one hour of sheer bliss! The centre also runs group 'get togethers', which cover everything from gentle yoga and qigong energy exercises to a special group for carers. If you have a problem, whether it is claiming benefits or trying to find holiday insurance, there is always someone who can give sensible advice and information.

Across Britain there are centres set up by organizations, such as Macmillan (www.macmillan.org.uk or call Cancerline on 0808 808 2020), Maggie's (www.maggiescentres.org), Cancer Resource Centre and Breast Cancer Haven (www.breastcancerhaven.org.uk), that offer a welcome and help. So find your nearest centre and *go*! Macmillan even have mobile information centres that visit high streets, communities and events to bring free, confidential information and support to everyone.

There are fantastic centres attached to hospitals, such as Cancerkin (www. cancerkin.org.uk) housed at the Royal Free Hospital in London. The enthusiasm and goodwill wraps around you, and they are full of helpful information.

Life changes

However much you want to get back into your old life, sometimes this isn't possible. I worked as a travel writer, but as a journalist I thought I would take advantage of things that had happened to me. I changed direction and started to write about cancer. This shows that there are plenty of things out there you might have *never* thought of doing, but now feel you want to – like dragon boat racing! This is growing as a participation sport around the world – with over one hundred breast cancer survivor dragon boat racing teams around the world. Each month another country signs up to offer training and fun in this unusual team sport. In the USA, cancer survivors are getting together to take up bowling, and again I see this happening across the world. These kinds of team activities can be truly life-enhancing.

Exercise

Any form of exercise is a good way of improving your health and regaining the mobility you will have lost lying around waiting for treatment. Swimming, cycling, walking, running, gardening – do whatever takes your fancy, and you will be doing the best thing possible to conquer fatigue and keep cancer at bay.

Exercise won't stop cancer returning, but if you keep healthy, you have a far better chance of overcoming it if it returns.

Aerobic exercise can help speed the recovery process following chemotherapy. Four years ago one of London's private hospitals started a revolutionary Cancer Recovery Exercise Programme. It was set up by a young New Zealander, Matt Hickey, and was so successful that NICE asked for a presentation on his system, then another, and then another. Sadly, they still haven't made up their minds and given the go-ahead for this to be offered on the NHS.

For anyone who was lucky enough to be on the pilot programme, they said that he was straight-talking, incredibly helpful, and understood more about cancer and how our bodies react than anyone else they were likely to meet.

'As one of his pioneer guinea pigs, he gave me a set of instructions to be handed to my local physio department in an NHS hospital. There, the head honcho was so interested that instead of being put on the waiting list . . . she phoned to ask, "Can you come in on Friday afternoon? Then we can have the whole department to ourselves."'

Many private insurance companies will actually pay for you to go on one of these programmes, and it's certainly worth asking as they have seen the incredible benefits it gives, especially quicker recovery times.

Join a club

Swimming is excellent exercise, as is aqua aerobics, which really gets you moving. Nothing is too difficult or strenuous. Or you could also join a gym. For somewhere near you, log onto www.fia.org.uk/choose-a-gym.html for details of local facilities. There is a lot on the site about how exercise can help various conditions (under the Health and Activity tab). Or you could contact your local council about gym facilities near you.

Physiotherapy

Like exercise, physio will help enormously in most cases to get you fit again. A number of chartered physiotherapists in the UK work in oncology and palliative care. There are three main treatment routes if you are resident in the UK and wish to see a physiotherapist:

Via the NHS

You will need to make an appointment with your GP and ask to be referred to see a physiotherapist. Onward referral will be at his or her discretion but you can discuss how you think a physiotherapist could help you.

Via private practitioners

If you can pay for your own treatment, there are many physiotherapists across the UK offering treatment – either in dedicated physiotherapy and sports-injury clinics or in your own home. To find a local private practitioner, go to the Chartered Society of Physiotherapy (CSP), www.csp.org.uk or call 020 7306 6666. The physiotherapy practitioners listed there give details of their areas of expertise and you can ask about their understanding of cancer when you call.

The Organisation of Chartered Physiotherapists in Private Practice (OCPPP), an occupational group of the CSP for private practitioners, also have a listing service, www.physiofirst.org.uk, 01604 684960. You can specify the area of practice required when you do your search online or ask when you call.

Via the independent sector

Some large employers run occupational health schemes for their employees. These may include provision for physiotherapy treatment. Check with your human resources or personnel department to see if you may be eligible. Private medical insurance schemes will often include physiotherapy treatment. Check with the scheme providers for eligibility, and ask whether they can provide a physiotherapist with an understanding of cancer.

It is also possible to access physiotherapy treatment through less common routes such as charities and the voluntary sector. If you do see a physiotherapist for private treatment, make sure they are chartered.

Mammograms

You will still need these, and your doctor will probably expect you to have these for the next five years – but private patients are monitored for ten years. If you feel you want a mammogram – ask.

Your secret life

Surprisingly, many patients say, *'Cancer was one of the best things that ever happened to me.'* All of a sudden, you are forced to look at your life, analyze what is important, and get rid of a lot of things you were doing out of duty. Cancer gives you a wonderful excuse to rid yourself of unwanted commitments, and do what you feel is best for you, your family and your friends. So now get out and enjoy life. You've worked hard to get this far – and you're worth it.

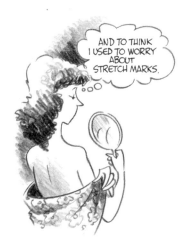

Chapter 18

Further information and contacts

Organizations and websites

These are all English-language websites that friends from round the world have found useful. Cancer is an international disease, after all.

American Association for Cancer Research (AACR) **www.aacr.org**
  This is the world's oldest and largest professional organization dedicated to advancing cancer research.
American Cancer Society (ACS) **www.cancer.org**
American Society of Breast Disease **www.asbd.org**
Asian Women's Breast Cancer Support Group **www.awbcg.co.uk**
Association for International Cancer Research (AICR) **www.aicr.org.uk**
Association of Cancer Online Resources **www.acor.org**
  A very helpful American site with information on clinical trials, books and survivor stories, etc.
Australian National Breast and Ovarian Cancer Centre **www.nbocc.org**
Betterdays Cancer Care **www.betterdays.uk.com**
  A UK organization that was set up to provide advocacy and support for women with breast cancer.

Breast Cancer Care **www.breastcancercare.org.uk** 0808 800 6000

Breastcancer.org **www.breastcancer.org**

British Complementary Medical Association **www.bcma.co.uk**
0845 345 5977

British Medical Association **www.bma.org.uk/ethics/health_records/AccessHealthRecords.jsp**

If you need to see your medical records, and find medics are being obstructive, remind them everyone is entitled to view their own health records. All competent patients may apply for access to their records under the 'Access to Health Records Act 1990' and the "Data Protection Act of 1998'

Canadian Breast Cancer Network **www.cbcn.ca**

Canadian Cancer Society **www.cancer.ca**

There is an excellent section on cancer myths and how unfounded they are.
If you receive a 'scare e-mail', go on to the Canada-wide page and click on 'About Cancer'. There is a link to 'Cancer Myths' on the left-hand side.

Cancer Council Australia **www.cancer.org.au**

Cancer.net **www.cancer.net**

Oncologist-approved and up-to-date cancer information from the American Society of Clinical Oncology.

Cancer Research UK **www.cancerresearchuk.org**

This is one of the most sensible and useful sites, with accurate and helpful day-to-day information, and rated worldwide. They have a very good helpline, 0808 800 4040 or 020 7121 6699. They also have useful information on **www.cancerhelp.org.uk** *and you can find out about clinical trials here. There is also an interesting free newsletter that you can subscribe to by applying by e-mail to cancer.spotlight@cancer.org.uk*

Cancersymptoms.org **www.cancersypmtoms.org**

A website sponsored by the Oncology Nursing Society that provides information to patients and caregivers about managing ten cancer treatment-related symptoms – anorexia, cognitive dysfunction, depression, dyspnoea, fatigue, hormonal disturbances, neutropenia, pain, peripheral neuropathy, and sexual dysfunction.

Department of Health UK **www.dh.gov.uk**

There are publications, information and key cancer policy documents on this website, such as the NHS Cancer Plan and the Manual of Cancer Standards.

Dr Susan Love Research Foundation **www.dslrf.org**
A research foundation that works to eradicate breast cancer and improve the quality of women's health through research, education, and advocacy.

Europa Donna: European Breast Cancer Coalition **www.europadonna.org**
An independent, non-profit organization whose members are affiliated groups from 42 European countries. The Coalition works to raise awareness of breast cancer and represents the interests of European women to local and national authorities, as well as to institutions of the European Union.

France – Cancer Support France **www.cancersupportfrance.info**
A very helpful website set up for English-speaking visitors or residents in France.

General Council for Massage Therapies **www.gcmt.org.uk** 0151 430 8199

Having Fun After Cancer **www.after-cancer.com**
My own website that gives more information about handling side effects, and dealing with life after treatment has finished.

Health Spa News **www.healthspanews.com**
Information for patients about travelling, holidays and where to find helpful hotels after treatment finishes.

Inflammatory Breast Cancer Help and Support **www.ibcsupport.org**

Inflammatory Breast Cancer Research Foundation **www.ibcresearch.org**
They provide e-mail discussion lists, an e-newsletter, volunteers who answer questions submitted to the website, articles, research information, videos, presentations, and inspirational stories on IBC.

Institute of Cancer Research **www.icr.ac.uk**
It has accurate information about the latest news and research.

Jules Bordet Institute, Belgium **www.bordet.be**
One of the most famous cancer treatment and research centres in the world.

Look Good, Feel Better **www.lookgoodfeelbetter.co.uk** or
www.lookgoodfeelbetter.com if outside the UK

Lymphoedema Support Network **www.lymphoedema.org** 020 7351 4480

Macmillan Cancerline **www.macmillan.org.uk** 0808 808 2020
You can find the nearest of 800 contact centres across the UK here.

Marie Curie Cancer Care **www.mariecurie.org.uk** 0800 716146

> *One of the most helpful organizations, and also one of the UK's largest charities. It provides care to around 27,000 terminally ill patients, with support for their families. They run a marvellous helpline that answers a wide range of queries.*

National Cancer Institute, USA **www.cancer.gov**

> *The following pages are particularly helpful:* **www.cancer.gov/cancertopics/ factsheet/Sites-Types/IBC** *and* **www.cancer.gov/cancertopics/pdq/ treatment/breast**.

National Center for Complementary and Alternative Medicine **nccam.nih.gov**

NHS **www.nhs.uk**

> *Information about the NHS: what it does, how it works, and how to use it. It also provides links through to other NHS organizations and local services.*

NICE (National Institute for Health and Clinical Excellence) **www.nice.org.uk**

> *The organization that has to approve drugs before they can be supplied by NHS.*

Quackwatch **www.quackwatch.com**

Factsheets, articles and publications

Breast Cancer Care has a large library of books. They are happy to look these out for you, if you contact the library team first and tell them what you want: libraryteam@breastcancercare.org.uk or call 0845 092 0838.

Macmillan produces a vast range of fact sheets and helpful booklets, including *Help with the Cost of Cancer*. Every cancer patient should have this useful free booklet, particularly if you have high transport expenses. It gives lots of information about getting these expenses paid. Call 0800 500 800.

Paul D'Auria Cancer Support Centre publish a range of booklets, including *Understanding and Living with Cancer, After Treatment – Physical Wellbeing* and *After Treatment – Emotional Wellbeing*. Call 020 7924 3924 to order copies. www.pauldauriacentre.org.uk.

Inflammatory Breast Cancer: a Canadian survivor's story

> www.abcn.ca/artman2/publish/Sharing_Our_Stories_22/ Inflammatory_Breast_Cancer_A_survivor_s_Story.html

Books

Please don't think you have to rush out and buy any of these – except perhaps one of Christine Beckwith Smith's humorous books. She has a marvellous website, and has published several books with hilarious cartoons about what we go through. www.cancerclub.com.

Even the Eyebrows? by Sharon Morrison (AuthorHouse, ISBN 978-1-4389-2334-5). If you are having problems with side effects you will love this, as Sharon graphically describes what happened to her. Mark out suitable lines and shove them under your consultant's nose when they say, "I've never heard of this before."

The Secret History of a Woman Patient by Janet Rhys Dent (Radcliffe Publishing, ISBN 978-1-84619-150-3)

Healing, Hype or Harm? Edzard Ernst (editor) (Imprint Academic, ISBN 978-1-84540118-4)

The Oxford Handbook of Complementary Medicine by Edzard Ernst, Max H Pittler, Barbara Wider, Kate Boddy (Oxford University Press, ISBN 978-0-19-920677-3)

Trick or Treatment by Simon Singh and Edzard Ernst (Bantam Press, ISBN 978-0-59306-129-9)

Newsletters and chatlines

Most charities send out newsletters, but here are the notable ones.

Cancerwire info@cancermonthly.com

American Association for Cancer Research has a zippy, informative online magazine aimed at survivors www.crmagazine.org/Pages/default.aspx

Talking Cancer is a website where patients and carers share their experiences of cancer and offer each other support. It seems to be read by Australian nurses (with expert knowledge) as well as the general public. There are a range of discussion forums covering general cancer topics, specific cancers, and support for carers. The forums provide the opportunity to connect with others online and you can read the forums freely. www.talkingcancer.org.

Overseas clinics

If you cannot obtain treatment in your own country, or if you are dissatisfied with your care, most people will contact one of the major cancer centres in America and Europe. Not only do they have fantastic research backing up their treatment, but they are very patient-focused.

M D Anderson's Clinic for women with IBC is believed to be the first such clinic in the world. The Inflammatory Breast Cancer Clinic accepts patients who are newly diagnosed or previously treated, and offers the most innovative treatments currently available. You can also view newsletters from MD Anderson's IBC programme on their site, www.mdanderson.org.

Dana Farber www.dana-farber.org. There is specific information for international patients.

Duke University Medical Center www.mc.duke.edu

John Hopkins www.hopkinsmedicine.org

Mayo Clinic www.mayoclinic.org

Memorial Sloane-Kettering www.mskcc.org

Washington Medical Center www.uwmedicine.org

Ludwig Institute for Cancer Research (worldwide) www.licr.org

Institut Gustave Roussy (France) www.igr.fr

Universitätsklinikum Jena (Germany) www.med.uni-jena.de

Centre Hospitalier Universitaire Saint-Pierre (Belgium) www.stpierre-bru.be

Hôpital Erasme (Cliniques Universitaires de Bruxelles) (Belgium) www.erasme.ulb.ac.be

Healthcare in Europe for UK citizens

Legislation is currently going through the European Parliament that will entitle UK citizens, in certain circumstances, to access healthcare in Europe if it can't be obtained in the UK, or if the wait is too long. For the latest information go to www.europarl.europa.eu/oeil/file.jsp?id=5661632 or the Public Health Portal of the European Union at http://ec.europa.eu/health-eu/care_for_me and click on the 'Mobility in Europe' tab. For more information on healthcare abroad go to http://ec.europa.eu/social/main.jsp?catId=509&langId=en.

Cancer support centres

Across Britain there are organizations that offer a warm welcome and a lot of help. If you haven't visited a cancer centre, do find your nearest and GO. Here is a list of some, but there might be others nearer to you.

Breast Cancer Haven (Fulham and Hereford) www.breastcancerhaven.org.uk

Barnet and District Cancer Link, North London There are Wednesday drop-in clinics at Catholic Church of Mary Immaculate, Union Street, Barnet (1.30–4 pm). Phone Eve on 020 8446 3104. They supply physiotherapy, reflexology, manicures, etc., but expect a waiting list!

Cancerkin, North London A unique breast cancer centre, based at the Royal Free Hospital, just off Hampstead Heath. 'Treat the patient, not just the cancer' has always been their maxim. The meetings are lively, full of fun, and offer lots of sensible information. Patients are referred from 35 hospitals within the London region to take advantage of their range of services. Whether you've just been diagnosed with breast cancer and want more information, or you're undergoing treatment and need some TLC, or you're caring for someone with breast cancer, Cancerkin's dedicated team is on hand to support you and your family. Contact them on 020 7830 2323 or 2310, www.cancerkin.org.uk, or e-mail info@cancerkin.org.uk.

Chelsea and Westminster Hospital, Southwest London A small but very welcoming information centre, with a limited amount of therapies, lots of sensible books and leaflets, and tea and coffees. Ground Floor, 369 Fulham Road, Chelsea, London SW10 9NH, 020 8237 2386, www.chelwest.nhs.uk.

Cherry Lodge Cancer Care, North London 23 Union Street, Barnet, EN5 4HY, 020 8441 7000, www.cherrylodgecancercare.org.uk.

Chrysalis, Surrey This is the Crawley Breast Cancer group who meet at 7.30pm every last working Monday of the month, at the Postgraduate Medical Centre, Crawley Hospital, West Green, Crawley. www.chrysalisbreastgroup.org.uk

Macmillan, UK-wide Marvellous centres all over Britain. Go to www.macmillan.org.uk and click on the 'How We Can Help' tab to find a centre near you. Or you can call 0808 808 00.

Maggie's Cancer Caring Centres, Scotland, London, Oxford, southwest Wales and Lanarkshire. Other centres to open soon. To find if there is a centre near you, go to www.maggiescentres.org or call 0131 537 2456.

Mulberry Centre, Middlesex. This is open every day, with late evenings four times a month. It offers a range of services including complementary therapies, workshops and information. West Middlesex University Hospital, Twickenham Road, Isleworth, TW7 6AF www.themulberrycentre.co.uk 020 8321 6300.

Paul D'Auria Cancer Centre, Southwest London This is the oldest of centres. Very welcoming and lots going on. Woburn House, 155-157 Falcon Road, London, SW11 2PD, www.pauldauriacentre.org.uk, 020 7924 3924.

Peterborough Breast Cancer Support Group A very go-ahead team with a lovely welcoming attitude. They meet on the first Thursday of each month at the Holiday Inn, Thorpe Wood Road, Peterborough between 8–10pm. www.peterboroughbreastcancersupportgroup.co.uk. Call 01780 720793.

Pinkladies Breast Cancer Support Group, Guernsey They get up to all sorts of fun things! www.pinkladies.org.gg, 07781 415131.

St. Mary's, Paddington Vicky Harmer runs a 'fun centre' with lots going on, and the nice thing is, if you have been treated at a London hospital with no centre, you are welcome to come here. 020 7886 1425.

Northern Ireland

The Ulster Cancer Foundation, Belfast Patient information conferences, support group meetings, counselling, art therapy, a mastectomy and head-wear fitting service, a family support service... The activities are impressive. You can call in for a chat to 40–44 Eglantine Avenue, Belfast BT9 6DX or call the helpline 0800 783 3339.

Cancer Lifeline 44 Alliance Avenue, Belfast, BT14 7PJ 028 90 351 999.

Cancer Choices 29 Carland Road, Dungannon, Co. Tyrone, BT71 4AA.

Care for Cancer 10 Prospect Court, Omagh, Co. Tyrone, BT78 1AR, 028 82 246 599.

LILAC 3 Barrack Square, Coalisland, Co. Tyrone, BT71 4JG, 028 87 746 600.

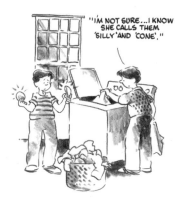

Chapter 19
Hero products

This is the 'advertising' section, where I shamelessly name commercial products that have been developed to help you. When medical professionals say, 'We are not allowed to recommend commercial products,' my response is 'So why did you recommend X drug, which is giving me so many problem side effects?' Drug companies are the most commercial and profitable companies in the world, so I find it weird that they are happy to prescribe drugs, but won't tell you about commercial products that can make drug side effects bearable.

When tamoxifen threw up horrible side effects for me, nurses and doctors just shrugged their shoulders and said they couldn't help. One nurse even peeled off layers of skin, saying, 'You do have a problem, but there is nothing I can advise.' It is no wonder that in Britain such a high percentage of patients elect to come off these drugs – and therefore don't have the advantage of the hormonal drug to help prevent cancer returning.

Being obstinate, I determined there must be solutions. After e-mailing major skincare companies, such as Clarins, Clinique and Estée Lauder, I was astonished by their knowledge of what I was going through. Yes, their research chemists knew all about the horrible things these drugs did to our skin. They had developed creams and products that would help.

So here are the secrets and names of companies that seriously help us with our problems. I have also included a little information about the company's history and how they developed their products. This is to show that these companies have teams of dedicated professionals behind their products.

As I have said before, I am NOT medically qualified, and can only tell you what has worked for me and friends. So before trying anything:

- Ask your doctor or nurse if the product is suitable.
- Ask the skincare consultant in store for a patch test (when they put a small sample on your arm – leave it 24 hours to see if you are allergic).
- Although many products say they are 'pure', 'botanical', 'organic', 'use fresh ingredients' etc, any company can use these 'buzz' words in advertising, and do. To use 'organic' the product may only have a tiny percentage of organic products, so the best guarantee that something is organic is to see if it has been approved by the Soil Association.
- However, there are excellent products (some of them having gone through clinical trials) that use certain chemicals in the ingredients. Every skincare product must have some preservative, otherwise it will soon go off. Your best guarantee is to see if it is approved by a food and drug agency or if it has been clinically trialled.

Skincare

Avene, www.avene.co.uk

This is one of the best-known French skin medical spa treatment centres, and although they specialize in treating other skin problems, cancer patients have been using their superb products very successfully.

Avene are particularly good at producing **gentle exfoliants** – their facial product and their body exfoliant are not only very gentle, but get rid of dry, flaky skin. Use these at least once a week to slough off dead skin, and encourage 'clean' skin to grow.

Clarins, uk.clarins.com

Clarins was one of the first companies to start using plants and plant extracts in their creams. Jacques Courtin-Clarins was passionate about good skin care, and drove his company forward to become one of the best-known in this field.

Today, **Clarins oils**, containing 100 per cent pure plant extracts, have been an unprecedented success, and one of their most popular products is its **Anti-Pollution Complex**, derived mainly from active plant ingredients.

Clinique, www.clinique.co.uk

Clinique were the first company to e-mail me about my horrible skin problems – yes, they were well aware of problems caused by drugs, and they had developed special creams to help patients! They take stands at dermatology and other medical conferences to tell the medical profession about them.

Their **Deep Comfort Body Butter** is excellent at restoring drug-dried skin after treatment. Their **Turnaround Facial Mask** is what I turn to when my face looks sallow and lifeless.

They have an excellent booklet (written for the medical profession) *Physicians' Guide to Clinique Products,* which lists every ingredient in their recommended skincare range, so staff can check if anything might produce a reaction to certain drugs.

Dr Bragi, www.dr.bragi.com

Dr Bragi's **Age Management Marine Enzyme**. This product is ace. It doesn't feel like a serum but it acts in the same way – instant First Aid for drug-stressed skin. I love the clear bottles filled with little air bubbles; these are genuine, part of the ingredients developed by this doctor from Iceland. The marine enzymes protect our skin from free radicals. It is an extremely effective product, but it is sensitive to lipids, so wait about 15 minutes before you apply any creams or foundations on top.

Estée Lauder, www.esteelauder.co.uk

This company is particularly strong in anti-ageing products, and in helping with dry skin problems. They were one of the first companies to produce serums, and have a helpful range that includes a **pore minimiser** (when drugs give you horrid open pores on your face), and several helpful night 'repair' serums.

Estée Lauder calls serums 'one of the greatest skincare innovations of all time' and, for once, I don't think this is media-hype. Serums look like nothing – you can't feel them on your face, but use them and your friends tell you how well you look. If I have strong drugs to take, I will use them twice a day, but otherwise once is enough, at night underneath your night cream.

Estée Lauder's **Advanced Night Repair** has been out for over 25 years, but is still going strong, and really lives up to its name. I used it twice a day after a major operation, when I was on about 20 different drugs, and friends thought I had been in hospital for a face lift! At £32 a bottle it is cheaper than most.

As one of the largest skincare companies in the world, this is a stalwart of the *Look Good, Feel Better* programme (www.lookgoodfeelbetter.co.uk), owning companies such as Clinique, Origins, Prescriptives, etc, who supply many of the products in our 'goodie boxes'. The company is passionate about their Breast Cancer Awareness Campaign, and raises millions for research each year.

Evolife www.myevolife.co.uk

This is a new kid on the block, but already used in many French hospitals. Originally the products were developed for psoriasis patients, but an alert medic transferred over to oncology, and found the Evolife products equally helpful – and that's how they started in the cancer sector. The range includes **Evoskin** for dry face and body skin, **Evonail** for cracked and broken nails, **Evomuncy** for mouth ulcers, **Evodry** for dry mouth, **Evocapil** for sensitive and itchy scalp, and the deoderent **Evodeo**.

La Roche Posay www.laroche-posay.uk

This is now an international skincare company. Its thermal spa is a massive medical complex treating over 8,000 patients a year, and the skincare range was developed for these patients. Its products are sold through dermatologists and chemists worldwide. La Roche Posay makes a special effort to provide suitable products for black and asian skin. **Anthelios** is recommended for people with black skin, those who have vitiligo, and is for every skin type that is photosensitive or photosensitive as a consequence of photosensitizing drugs (chemotherapeutic drugs are known photosensitizers). Also, people with black skin who require camouflage make-up post-procedure or as a consequence of a skin pathology can use the **Unifiance range** of make-up (available in most countries that stock LRP including Ireland, but not the UK, so those in Britain have to order it on the net). They don't, however, have a range specifically developed for black skin. The **Toleriane range** is also especially suitable for 'cancer drug skins', and the company has carried out 21 clinical trials of its products. If you or your doctor wants copies, go on their website and send an e-mail.

iS Clinical, www.isclinical.com

A new American company that has hit the UK market. iS Clinical's products have been tested in clinical trials in the USA. The company participates in philanthropic programmes for the benefit of cancer patients suffering from radiation and chemotherapy treatments, acne patients, and burn patients. One such programme was initiated at the Washington Cancer Institute in Washington D.C. in early 2003, and has been tremendously successful. You may never have heard of the company, but they are the philanthropic off-shoot of Mentor, the company that makes prostheses.

Their **Body Complex** is a brilliant skin cream; they call it 'innovative skincare' and it really is. At the Washington Institute, women use this twice a day – reducing to once a day when their skin feels 'normal'. The other products are also extremely helpful, particularly their **serums**. And if you really want a lift, apparently the facial they developed, **Fire and Ice**, has become a 'beauty secret' of stars such as Gwyneth Paltrow. Fire and Ice is coming to salons in the UK, and if you go on their website you will see where it is becoming available.

Sisley, www.sisley-cosmetics.co.uk

This is another French company that quietly gets on with making excellent (but expensive) products. Their little jar of **Lip Balm** is a lifesaver for dried-up lips. Their **All Day All Year** serum works whenever you need an extra skin boost, and the **Confort Extreme** night cream is a skin-saver when drugs have done their worst on your face.

Udderly Smooth www.udderlysmooth.co.uk

A crew member on a round-the-world yacht race discovered Udderly Smooth in the USA, and what's good for sea-battered skin is also very helpful for cancer patients. Two comments on the websites says it all:

> 'I started using Udderly Smooth after searching for an excellent skin cream, because I am having radiotherapy and chemotherapy. Udderly Smooth is just the ticket, as my skin is sensitive at the best of times, and my friend recommended it as they use it in the States for patients. We need to get this on the NHS as a first choice of creams to be used. Please, please! Works a treat!'

> 'I had breast cancer a couple of years ago and wear a prosthesis as a result. The prosthesis makes my scar very sore . . . A friend in the support group recommended Udderly Smooth to soothe and prevent irritation, so, doubting it, I tried some. I was so impressed! It took away perhaps 95 per cent of the irritation and it continues to improve all the time! Love it!'

Weleda, www.weleda.co.uk

Way back in Celtic times, wise women, or Weledas, looked after the sick and injured. These were women with a deep knowledge of nature, and today their name lives on in a line of natural skincare products that are often helpful for cancer patients.

They make a very good **Almond Skincare range** (fragrance-free and formulated for skin that is super-sensitive, easily upset or very dry): **Almond Intensive Facial Cream** (rich and creamy), **Almond Cleansing Lotion**, **Almond Facial Oil** (protective, soothing, nourishing facial oil) and **Almond Facial Masque** (soothing masque to boost skin radiance). Or there is their **Calendula** baby range, which only contains very gentle non-skin-stimulating essential oils, and soothing plant extracts, and has been dermatologically-tested on skin that is prone to eczema and dermatitis.

Barefoot Botanicals, www.barefoot-botanicals.com

Homeopaths Jonathan Stallick and Hilery Dorrian have created Barefoot Botanicals to help people with problem skins. One of their most helpful ranges is the **Rosa Fina** range. They say the secret of their success lies in advanced formulations, which combine the cutting-edge science with a thousand years of herbal wisdom. Ingredients are carefully sourced to provide performance with therapeutic benefits. The **S.O.S Skin Rescue** range has been designed for especially dry skin and is also suitable for those suffering with eczema, psoriasis and dermatitis.

Champneys, www.champneys.com

The well-known health farm has turned to producing skincare products. Trying them out, I was struck by the 'nice feel' they gave my face, and wanting to know more, was told this was thanks to isoflavones, active compounds from soybeans. They make very good **hand and nail creams**, and **body lotions** – and what I love, a **Body Glistening Oil**.

Finders, www.findershealth.com or www.shopforspa.com

When I went to the Klinic Bad Sulza in Germany, I found they were using products from this company, and it is British! So this proves they are ace!

Once your skin has healed, you should try a body scrub once a week: the sort with oil in it. It gets rid of rough patches, feeds your skin, and sets it up to absorb and renew itself. Finders makes one of the best, called **Salt Brushing**, and it is under £10.

The same company also makes **Black Mud Mask Soap**, which prevents your hands drying out when washing. And, to add to their helpful products, their **Dead Sea Spa Magik Hair Magic Serum** is fantastic for hair.

Floris, www.florislondon.com

J. Floris Ltd is now run by the eighth generation descendants of its founder and still trades out of the original premises at 89 Jermyn Street. They continue to use many unique practices, including one dating from when Floris first began to accept cash payments. It was considered extremely bad form to give customers dirty or crumpled change, so all coins were scrubbed clean and notes were pressed flat. The customer's change would then be produced, clean and sparkling, on a velvet covered mahogany change-pad – thus ensuring that neither staff nor customer would suffer the embarrassment of their hands touching or ladies' gloves getting dirty. Today, customers are still handed their change in this manner, although the practice of 'laundering' money has disappeared!

Since opening in 1730, Floris has had many famous customers, including Florence Nightingale, Mary Shelley, Beau Brummell, and Ian Fleming (the 'real' James Bond), a regular customer who always wore Floris No. 89.

Floris has an incredible range of bath and body products, all with lovely floral scents, and all very mild so that you can use them.

Hair

If you lose your hair completely, there are many charities that can help, and hospitals are getting better at supplying wigs. Charles Worthington is a wonderful person, founder of the eponymous hair salons, and a stalwart of the *Look Good, Feel Better* programme. His salons have dedicated stylists who just love to get their fingers into an NHS wig and transform it. Until you have seen what magic they work with their scissors you wouldn't believe what can be done.

If you don't lose your hair, the side effects of drugs can still cause very dry, 'straw hair' and 'fish hooks hair'. This is when it is actually painful to drag a brush or comb through your hair. Under a microscope you can see that the hair has split all along the shaft, leaving bits that catch in everything. When I asked PD (pompous dermatologist) what could I do about it, he told me to 'Use a conditioner'. Really! Cancer-stressed hair needs something strong, so another 'expert' was deleted from my book, and I went looking.

Tara Smith

I was lucky to meet up with bubbly Tara Smith. When people talk about 'hairdresser to the stars', Tara is the genuine article. Her hair shampoos and conditioners are wonderful and readily available. www.tarasmith.com.

Schwarzkopf

They make a **GLISS** range which is excellent. There is the usual shampoo and conditioner, but their secret weapon is a spray-on shine – brilliant.

For straw hair, there is a new product range called **Biolustré.** They have an **Exfoliating Shampoo**, which you use at first to strip away old shampoo residue, and any 'nasties' that might be leaching from the drugs. Then use the **Treatment Shampoo**, and after the **Daily Conditioning Sealant**. This range gets top marks from all who have tried the range.

Finders, www.findershealth.com
Another excellent hair range is the **Dead Sea Spa Magik** range, made by Finders. Their range includes a **Mineral Shampoo** (which also helps if you have dandruff), a **Conditioning Scalp Mud** which helps with itchy scalp, and the brilliant **Hair Magic Serum** – which you can use like a conditioner – or if your hair is really bad, comb it through before you dry your hair, and leave on.

John Bell and Croyden, www.johnbellcroyden.co.uk
After my meeting with PD and seething from frustration, I stumped along Wigmore Street, and came across a sign 'Free Advice – Trichology Clinic' in the window of the chemists John Bell and Croyden. What had I got to lose? Well, Vanessa soon showed she was made of more intelligent stuff than PD. Examining my hair carefully, she said it was a clear case of damage from tamoxifen, and gave me three products; treatment cream, shampoo and conditioner. They cost around £100 for a three month's supply but they were worth every penny as the fish hooks disappeared. Now I 'mix and match' depending on my budget, and my hair is almost back to its old shine.

Hair colour

A friend ended up with grey hair after chemo, even though she is much too young, but didn't dare colour it because of bad experiences in the past. Another friend recommended Karine Jackson's Hair and Beauty salon in the centre of London. Karine is one of those lovely bubbly enthusiasts whom you want to hug and trust immediately. She has studied the effects of cancer drugs on our hair, and is working with others to try and develop a network of hairdressers across Britain who understand how to combat drug side effects. She has teamed up with Organic Colour Systems, whose products contain far less of the harmful chemicals, and substitute natural products whenever possible.

If you go to www.karinejackson.co.uk the site gives prices, which are incredibly low, if you take into account the quality of care and the enjoyment you get from the experience.

Hands

Cancer drugs often cause the top layer of nails to flake off, which can be painful as nails catch in clothes. You might suddenly find your hands and feet develop horrid horny nails, and splitting skin, and you can almost see your fingernails disintegrating. You may feel it is trivial and silly to make a fuss about this, but don't! These are important parts of our body, and wouldn't be there if they were just for decoration. The Oncolink (the website of a cancer centre in the USA) has a useful *Nail and Skin Care Tip Sheet*. It is a bit patronising, but at least they are trying! www.oncolink.com/coping/article.cfm?c=5&s=75&ss=186&id=991.

Of course you WILL use rubber gloves, won't you? That is probably the single-most important facet of hand care. Having said that, you will find that drugs make your hands incredibly rough – but there are helpful products:

Clarins

Their **Hand and Nail Treatment Cream** is one of the best on the market. I understand even the Queen uses it!

NailTek® www.nailtek.com

The Royal Marsden Hospital used to have a manicurist, Francesca Manning, who was very helpful and supportive. She made me realize that many others suffer – usually in silence. One thing Francesca recommended was NailTek® products, made in the USA for cancer patients. They have **Crystal Glass Files**, soft and gentle and so good I have one by the bed, in my handbag and on my desk – all places where the horrid little hangnails catch.

NailTek® also make special base coats. The best one for splitting and hang nails is **Hydration Therapy II** (a nail varnish). If you have horrid thick, horny nails, then their **Hydration Therapy III** is the right product. They also make **Cuticle Crème** and **NailTek Renew**; products which feed the nails, and really help them grow again.

Provided I remember to use their Hydration Therapy clear nail varnish every day, and their cuticle cream at night, my nails now have a white edge – before they were like a serrated saw.

Feet

Fiona is a very practical Practice Manager at my local GPs. One of her tips for cracked feet or hands is to mix a couple of capfuls of **baby oil** with good-quality **lavender oil**, tip a good splodge into a bowl of warm water, and sit with your feet in this for 20 minutes. As she says, lavender is antiseptic and stops infection, the oils are healing, and it smells lovely!

Another of her tips is to eat **manuka honey** (Rowse make a very pure one) – or you can do as they do in New Zealand and spread it on broken skin. Ask advice first, but it is one of nature's healers.

Shuropody www.shuropody.com

Shuropody is a footcare retailer with around 60 chiropody/podiatry salons around the UK, from Aberdeen to Plymouth. If you have cracked, painful skin on your feet, they have a special **Intensive Repair Cream**, and gadgets to get rid of 'build-up' of skin, corns, etc. The salons offer reflexology too, so you can really have a pampering session, before floating out into the world! And a lovely tip for summer – blast hot feet with the cold-air setting on your hairdryer.

Once you have gorgeous feet, keep them that way! After any bath or shower, pat feet dry and rub in cream. Clinique have a **Water Treatment** cream which is wonderful and Barefoot Botanicals make lovely citrus-smelling **Foot Balm**. But I have found that **Flexitol** (on NHS prescription) is also very good, and as most people can get this free on prescription in England and Wales, it is worth asking for. For some reason it is only included on one NHS approval list, but just tell doctors to keep looking: they'll find it eventually.

If cold feet or swollen ankles are a problem, try Charnos' **Cotton Modal Tights** – modal being a lovely, soft fibre made out of reconstituted cellulose from beech trees. They aren't as bulky as wool, but are just as warm.

Sun protection

We MUST protect our faces at all times, even when we go out in the winter – skin cancer is on the rise, and effects of hormonal drugs give us 'brillo pad' skin. The companies previously mentioned, particularly La Roche Posay with their Anthelios range, Clinique, Clarins, and Estée Lauder, all make excellent suncare products. Make sure you slap it on, and do this 15 minutes before you go in to the sun. Let it soak in – don't rub it in, as this gives better protection.

Itching

This can drive you mad, but a novel way of alleviating the itching is applying an **Ice Bandage** (www.icebandage.co.uk), normally used for sports injuries. It comes in a sleek, silver pack containing a moist, soft bandage which cools the site for up to two hours. Cooling the site has a counter-irritant effect.

Don't ever think you are being vain to seek help with skin problems. Our skin is vitally important to us. If it is cracked and diseased it will let in germs and other nasties, and could cause more problems. So cherish your skin – it's the only one you have!

Glossary

This glossary includes words, acronyms and terms that you might come across on your cancer journey. Many of the definitions come from the National Cancer Institute's on-line dictionary at www.cancer.gov,. They have over 400 definitions under 'A' alone!

A

acute A sudden onset of symptoms or disease.

adenoma A benign tumour made up of glandular tissue. For example, an adenoma of the pituitary gland may cause it to produce abnormal amounts of hormones.

adjuvant chemotherapy *see* **chemotherapy**

adverse effect An unwanted side effect of treatment.

AFP (alpha fetoprotein) A tumour marker.

aggressive A quickly growing cancer.

alendronate sodium A drug that affects bone metabolism. It is used in treating osteoporosis and Paget's disease and is being studied in the treatment of hypocalcaemia (abnormally high levels of calcium in the blood) and in treating and reducing the risk of bone pain caused by cancer. Alendronate sodium belongs to the family of drugs called bisphosphonates.

alternative medicine Practices not generally recognized by the medical community as standard or conventional medical approaches and used instead of standard treatments.

analgesics Drugs that reduce pain. These drugs include aspirin, acetaminophen and ibuprofen.

anastrozole An anti-cancer drug that belongs to the family of drugs called nonsteroidal aromatase inhibitors. Anastrozole is used to decrease oestrogen production and suppress the growth of tumours that need oestrogens to grow.

anaemia When you have less than the normal amount of red blood cells (haemoglobin) in the blood. This may be due to bleeding, lack of blood production by the bone marrow or to the brief survival of blood already manufactured. Symptoms include tiredness, shortness of breath and weakness.

anaesthesia Loss of feeling or awareness. Local anaesthetics cause loss of feeling in a part of the body. General anaesthetics put the person to sleep.

anaesthetics Substances that cause loss of feeling or awareness. Local anaesthetics cause loss of feeling in a part of the body. General anaesthetics put the person to sleep.

angiogram An X-ray of blood vessels; the person receives an injection of dye to outline the vessels on the X-ray.

antibiotic A drug used to treat infections caused by bacteria and other microorganisms.

antibody A type of protein made by certain white blood cells in response to a foreign substance (antigen). Each antibody can bind to only a specific antigen. The purpose of this binding is to help destroy the antigen. Antibodies can work in several ways, depending on the nature of the antigen. Some antibodies destroy antigens directly. Others make it easier for white blood cells to destroy the antigen.

antiemetics Drugs that prevent or reduce nausea and vomiting.

antivirals Drugs used to treat infections caused by viruses.

areola The area of dark-coloured skin on the breast that surrounds the nipple.

aspirate Fluid withdrawn from a lump, often a cyst, or a nipple.

aspiration Removal of fluid from a lump, often a cyst, with a syringe.

asymptomatic Having no signs or symptoms of disease.

auto-immune disease Condition in which the body recognizes its own tissues as foreign and directs an immune response against them.

auto-immunity Condition in which the body's immune system mistakenly fights and rejects the body's own tissues.

axilla The armpit. Lymph glands in the armpit are called the axilliary nodes. Certain cancers, such as breast cancer, spread to the axillary nodes. Axillary lymph nodes are usually removed by surgery to determine if breast cancer is present and if treatment with chemotherapy is necessary.

axillary Pertaining to the armpit area.

axillary dissection Surgery to remove lymph nodes found in the armpit.

axillary lymph node dissection Surgery to remove lymph nodes found in the armpit region.

axillary lymph nodes Lymph nodes found in the armpit that drain the lymph channels from the breast.

axillary nodes Lymph nodes – also called lymph glands – found in the armpit.

B

benign Not cancerous, not spreading, non-malignant.

benign growth A swelling or growth that is not cancerous and does not spread from one part of the body to another.

bilateral Both sides of the body.

biopsy The surgical removal of tissue for microscopic examination to aid diagnosis.

blood cells The red cells, white cells and platelets that make up the blood. They are made in the bone marrow.

blood count Examination of a blood specimen in which the number of white blood cells, red blood cells and platelets are determined.

bolus (or push) chemotherapy *see* **chemotherapy**

bone marrow The spongy material found inside the bones. Most blood cells are made in the bone marrow.

bone marrow biopsy and aspiration The procedure by which a needle is inserted into a bone to withdraw a sample of bone marrow.

bone marrow suppression A decrease in the production of blood cells. Sometimes, bone marrow suppression is a side effect of chemotherapy.

bone marrow transplant The infusion of bone marrow into a patient who has been treated with high dose chemotherapy or radiation therapy. Patients may use their own marrow, which in some cases has been frozen.

bone scan A picture of the bones using a radioactive dye that shows any injury, disease, or healing. This is a valuable test to determine if cancer has spread to the bone, if anti-cancer therapy has been successful, and if affected bony areas are healing.

breast prosthesis An artificial breast that fits inside a bra to replace all or part of a natural breast. Usually made from soft silicone gel encased in a thin film, moulded to form the natural shape of a woman's breast, or part of a breast.

BSE (breast self-examination) A manual self-examination of the breasts.

C

cancer A general term for more than 200 diseases characterized by the uncontrolled, abnormal growth of cells in different parts of the body, that can spread to other parts of the body.

cancer in situ The stage where the cancer is still confined to the tissue in which it started.

carcinogen A substance that causes cancer. For example, nicotine in cigarettes is a carcinogen that causes lung cancer.

carcinomas A form of cancer that develops in the tissues covering or lining organs of the body, such as the skin, uterus, lung or breast. Eighty to 90 percent of all cancers are carcinomas.

carcinoma in situ The earliest stage of cancer, in which the tumour is still confined to the local area, before it has grown to a significant size or has spread. In situ carcinomas are highly curable.

CAT scan (CT scan) A test using computers and x-rays to create images of various parts of the body.

catheter A tube made of rubber, plastic or metal that can be introduced into a body cavity to drain fluid or deliver fluids or medication.

CEA (carcinoembryonic antigen) A blood tumour marker.

central venous catheter A special intravenous tubing that is surgically inserted into a large vein near the heart and exits from the chest or abdomen. The catheter allows medications, fluids, or blood products to be given and blood samples to be taken.

chemotherapy The use of chemicals (drugs or medications) to kill malignant cells. Numerous drugs have been developed for this purpose and most act to injure the DNA of the cells. When the DNA is injured, the cells cannot grow or survive. Successful chemotherapy depends on the fact that malignant cells are somewhat more sensitive to the drugs than normal cells. Because the cells of the marrow, the intestinal tract, the skin and hair follicles are most sensitive to these drugs, injury to these organs cause the common side effects of chemotherapy (mouth sores, hair loss, etc). *Adjuvant chemotherapy* Chemotherapy used along with surgery or radiation therapy. It is usually used in cases where there is high risk of hidden cancer cells remaining and may increase the likelihood of cure by destroying small amounts of undetectable cancer. *Bolus (or push) chemotherapy* Administration of intravenous chemotherapy over a short time, usually five minutes or less. *Infusion chemotherapy* Treatment which may last from 15 minutes to several hours or days.

chronic Persisting over a long period of time.

clinical nurse specialist Does just what the title suggests – and very often more.. They are there to help guide cancer patients on their treatment path, and often lecture and inform other medical staff in a hospital about cancer and how they can work treating the disease.

colonoscopy A procedure to look at the colon or large bowel through a lighted, flexible tube.

clinical trials The procedure in which new cancer treatments are tested. The treatment is evaluated for its effectiveness in reducing or eliminating disease. A clinical trial may be done by a government agency, a drug company or a hospital to determine the most effective dose of a drug, to compare different combinations of treatments, or to determine the effect of the drug on a tumour.

consultant surgeon In teaching hospitals, consultants are often professors.

cycle of treatment Designates an intensive, clustered period of chemotherapy and/or radiation. The treatment may be given for several days or weeks, and represents one cycle of treatment. The treatment plan may call for two, three or more cycles of treatment.

cyst An accumulation of fluid or semi-solid material within a sac.

D

drug resistance The result of cells' ability to resist the effects of a specific drug. The development of resistance in cancer cells to a specific drug or drugs. If resistance develops, a patient in remission from chemotherapy may relapse despite continued administration of anticancer drugs.

dysphagia Difficulty in swallowing; a sensation of food sticking in the throat.

dyspnea Difficult or painful breathing; shortness of breath.

E

edema The accumulation of fluid in part of the body.

effusion A collection of fluid in a body cavity, usually between two adjoining tissues. For example, a pleural effusion is the collection of fluid between two layers of the pleura (the lung's covering).

electrolytes Certain chemicals – including sodium, potassium, chloride and bicarbonate, found in the tissues and blood. They are often measured as an aid to patient care.

erythema Red patches on the skin. Erythema of the skin may be a sign of underlying infection or inflammation. Chemotherapy injections may also cause erythema of the skin. This usually disappears within several hours. Persistent redness of the skin at a chemotherapy site should be brought to the attention of a nurse or doctor.

estrogen *see* **oestrogen**

excision Surgical removal.

extravasation Leakage into the surrounding tissues of intravenous fluids or drugs, especially cancer chemotherapeutic agents, from the vein being used for injection. Extravasation may damage the tissues.

F

fine-needle aspirate A procedure in which a needle is inserted, under local anaesthesia, to obtain a sample for the evaluation of suspicious tissue.

frozen section A technique in which tissue is removed by biopsy, then frozen, cut into thin slices, stained and examined under a microscope. A pathologist can rapidly examine a frozen section for an immediate diagnosis. This procedure is often done during surgery to help the physician decide the most appropriate course of action.

G

gamma-ray Electromagnetic radiation gamma rays are very high-energy electromagnetic rays that are sometimes used in cancer radiotherapy.

gene An organized sequence of bases on a chromosome that highlights the information necessary to construct a specific protein using the genetic code.

Every cell contains thousands of genes that act as blueprints to produce proteins that are essential to the cell's function.

gene therapy An experimental technique where normal genes are introduced into cells in place of missing or defective ones in order to correct genetic disorders.

genetic code The 'language' in which DNA's instructions are written. Every one of the 25,000 genes in each of our cells carries the information to make a single protein from amino acids. The sequence of bases along the gene specifies the sequence of amino acids in the protein.

genetic test A test that analyses the DNA in our cells to determine how those cells will behave. For example, women who have several relatives with breast cancer can have a test that will determine whether they have inherited a gene from their parents that makes them more susceptible to the disease.

gland An organ that makes and releases particular substances.

glandular tissue Tissue made up of cells that make and release something. Usually found lining the inside of an organ.

gynaecology Branch of medicine concerned with the functions and diseases specific to women and girls, especially those affecting the reproductive system.

H

haematology A branch of biology (physiology), pathology, clinical laboratory, internal medicine, etc, that is concerned with the study of blood, the blood-forming organs, and blood diseases. Blood diseases affect the production of blood and its components, such as blood cells, haemoglobin, blood proteins, the mechanism of coagulation, etc. The lab work is performed by a medical technologist.

haematologist A doctor who specializes in the problems of blood and bone marrow.

HER2 This stands for human epidermal growth factor receptor. It is a protein found in small amounts on normal breast cells. It is one of the proteins involved in cell growth. About a quarter of breast cancers have too much of this protein – they are said to be HER2 positive.

Herceptin® (trastuzumab) A type of targeted treatment for breast cancer. It is a monoclonal antibody, which means a single type of antibody that can be made in the laboratory in large quantities. Antibodies are molecules made naturally by our immune systems. Their role is to seek out foreign cells – bacteria and viruses for example – and kill them off. Antibodies made in the lab can be designed to seek out particular human cells. Herceptin® is designed to target breast cancer cells.

heredity The passing on of characteristics to the next generation via the genes. You can inherit physical or mental characteristics or the tendency to develop particular illnesses. Half your chromosomes (and so half your genes) come from your mother and half from your father.

high dependency unit A ward where you receive closer medical and nursing attention than on a regular ward. A high dependency unit typically has one nurse per patient or every two patients.

high-dose chemotherapy Anti-cancer drug treatment using very high drug doses. It is often followed by a transfusion of bone marrow or stem cells.

high-factor suncream A suncream that provides maximum protection against ultraviolet light. Cancer Research UK recommends using at least factor 15. This filters out 93 per cent of the sun's harmful rays. Factor 60 filters out 98 per cent.

high grade Means the cells look very different to normal cells. So the cancer may grow more quickly and be more likely to spread than low grade cancer.

histology The study of body tissues and cells. When a biopsy is 'sent for histology' it is looked at under a microscope to find the type of body tissue it is. If it is a cancer the laboratory does tests to see which type of cancer it is.

Hodgkin's disease A cancer that affects the lymph nodes. *See* **non-Hodgkin's lymphoma**.

hormonal drugs *see* **hormone therapy**

hormone Natural chemicals secreted by various organs of the body to regulate growth, metabolism, and reproduction. Some cancers are stimulated to grow by hormones, including the sex hormones (testosterone in men and oestrogen in women).

hormone dependent (hormone sensitive) A hormone dependent cancer is one that is stimulated to grow by the presence of a particular hormone. Breast cancer and prostate cancer can be hormone dependent cancers.

hormone replacement therapy (HRT) Treatment with sex hormones to replace those no longer being produced. Women may take oestrogen alone, or more usually, oestrogen and progesterone after natural or early menopause. Men may take testosterone after having both testicles removed during cancer treatment. HRT should not be taken by people with hormone dependent cancers.

hormone therapy (hormone treatment) Treating a disease with hormones, or by blocking the action of hormones, or surgical removal of hormone-producing glands to kill cancer cells or slow their growth. The most common hormonal therapy for breast cancer is the drug tamoxifen. Other hormonal therapies include megestrol, aminoglutethimide, androgens and surgical removal of the ovaries (oophorectomy). *See also* **tamoxifen.**

hospice A place where they care for patients who are terminally ill. The focus of hospice care is not to cure the patient but to improve the quality of life for whatever time the patient has left, and to make the dying process as comfortable and pain free as possible. Support is also offered to the patient's family members.

hot flushes A sudden feeling of being very hot. You may also go red in the face and sweat. It usually lasts for a few minutes. These effects occur in women going through the menopause or 'change of life'. They may also be caused by some cancer treatments in women and men.

I

immunity (immune system) The body's ability to fight infection and disease.

immunosuppression Weakening of the immune system that causes a lowered ability to fight infection and disease.

immunotherapy A treatment that stimulates the body's own defence mechanisms to combat disease, such as cancer.

indwelling catheter One type of catheter used with patients receiving chemotherapy and/or nutritional support. An indwelling catheter is a special tubing inserted into a large vein in the upper chest. The catheter is tunnelled under the skin of the chest to keep it firmly in place. The external end of the catheter can be used to administer medications, fluids, or blood products or to withdraw blood samples.

infiltration The leaking of fluid or medicines into tissues, which can cause swelling.

infusion Delivering fluids or medications into the bloodstream over a period of time.

infusion pump A device that delivers measured amounts of fluids or medications into the bloodstream over a period of time.

injection Pushing a medication into the body with the use of a syringe. *Intramuscular (IM) injection* into the muscle. *Intravenous (IV) injection* into the vein. *Subcutaneous injection* into the fatty tissue under the skin.

interferon A natural body protein produced by normal cells that is capable of killing cancer cells or stopping their unrestrained growth. Interferon was originally discovered as an antiviral agent, but has now been found to have some anti-cancer activity as well. Interferon may be artificially produced in large quantities using the technique of recombinant DNA.

in situ A very early stage of cancer when the tumour is localized to one area.

invasive cancer A stage of cancer in which cancer cells have spread to healthy tissue adjacent to the tumour.

L

lesion A lump or abscess possibly caused by injury or disease, such as cancer.

leukaemia Cancer of the blood. White blood cells may be produced in excessive amounts and are unable to work properly.

leukopenia A low number of white blood cells.

localized A cancer confined to the site of origin without evidence of spread.

lumpectomy Removal of a cancerous breast lump and the surrounding tissue without removing the entire breast. It is a less radical procedure than mastectomy and is usually followed by radiation treatment.

lymph angiogram A test to look at the lymph nodes.

lymphatic system A network that includes lymph nodes, lymph, and lymph vessels that serves as a filtering system for the blood.

lymphoedema Swelling, usually of an arm or leg, caused by obstructed lymphatic vessels. It can develop because of a tumour, or as an effect of surgery or radiation.

lymph node One of the many small, bean-shaped organs of the immune system linked by lymphatic vessels throughout the body. They make and store many different immune cells that fight infections.

lymphocytes White blood cells that kill viruses and defend against the invasion of foreign material.

M

malignant Cancerous. Two qualities of malignancies are the tendency to penetrate the tissues or organ, in which it originated, and to break off and spread elsewhere ('metastasize').

malignant tumour A tumour made up of cancer cells of the type that can spread to other parts of the body.

mammogram (mammography) A low-dose X-ray/picture of the breasts to determine whether abnormal growths or cysts are present.

mastectomy The surgical removal of the breast. *Segmental (lumpectomy)* is a removal of the lump and a small amount of surrounding breast tissue. *Simple (modified mastectomy)* is the removal of the entire breast. *Radical* is the removal of the entire breast along with underlying muscle and lymph nodes of the armpit.

melanoma A cancer of the pigment-forming cells of the skin or the retina of the eye.

metastasis The spread of cancer from one part of the body to another by way of the lymph system or bloodstream. Cells in the new tumour are like those in the original tumour.

monoclonal antibodies Artificially manufactured antibodies specifically designed to find targets on cancer cells for diagnostic or treatment purposes.

MRI (magnetic resonance imaging) This technique details images of body structures. It differs from a CT Scan in that the patient is not exposed to X-rays. The signals generated in the tissues in response to the magnetic field are converted by computer into images of body structures.

mucositis Inflammation of the mucous membranes. Soreness, like 'cold sores', can develop in the mouth as a side effect of chemotherapy.

myelosuppression A decrease in the production of red blood cells, platelets, and some white blood cells by the bone marrow.

N

nadir The lowest point to which white blood cell or platelet counts fall after chemotherapy.

neoplasm An abnormal growth or tumour.

neuropathy Malfunction of a nerve, often causing numbness (sensory nerve) or weakness (motor nerve). Sometimes a side effect of chemotherapy drugs.

neutropenia A blood condition characterized by the virtual absence of neutrophils, one type of white blood cell that is crucial to the body's defence against infection. Neutropenia can be caused by chemotherapy, radiation therapy or by cancer itself.

neutrophils A blood cell that fights infections. Often, it is not present in sufficient quantities in patients with acute leukaemia or after chemotherapy, which increases their susceptibility to infection.

nipple The tip of the breast; the pigmented projection in the middle of the areola. The nipple contains the opening of milk ducts from the breast. The nipple consists mainly of skin and ductal breast tissue.

nipple discharge Any fluid coming from the nipple. It may be clear, milky, bloody, tan, grey, or green.

nodule A small solid mass.

Non-Hodgkin's lymphoma A cancer of the lymphatic system. Non-Hodgkin's lymphoma is related to Hodgkin's disease but is made up of different cell types.

O

OCN (oncology certified nurse) A registered nurse who has met the requirements and successfully completed a certification examination in oncology.

oestrogen A female hormone secreted by the ovaries, which is essential for menstruation, reproduction and the development of secondary sex characteristics, such as breasts. Also known as estrogen.

oestrogen-receptor assay A test that determines whether the breast cancer in a particular patient is stimulated by oestrogen.

oncologist A physician who specialises in cancer therapy. Medical oncologists are internists with expertise in chemotherapy and the handling of general medical problems that arise during treatment of cancer. Radiation oncologists specialize in the use of radiation to treat cancer.

oncology The study and treatment of cancer. Doctors who specialize in oncology are called oncologists.

oncology clinical nurse specialist A registered nurse with a master's degree in oncology nursing who specializes in the care of cancer patients. Oncology nurse specialists may prepare and administer treatments, monitor patients, prescribe and provide supportive care, and teach and counsel patients and their families.

P

Paget's disease of the breast This can be confused with IBC, as many symptoms are the same. Nine out of ten women have an underlying breast cancer. The underlying breast cancer may be an invasive breast cancer or ductal carcinoma in situ (DCIS). Around half of the women who have Paget's disease will have a breast lump that can be felt at the time it is diagnosed. Paget's disease occurs in about one or two out of every 100 women with breast cancer. It usually occurs in women in their 50s, but can occur at a younger or older age. It can affect men. It usually first appears as a scaly, red rash affecting the nipple and sometimes the dark area of skin surrounding the nipple (the areola). The rash always affects the nipple first, and may then affect the areola. It does not go away and may become sore. The area may bleed slightly. Paget's disease can be confused with other skin conditions such as eczema, dermatitis or psoriasis, as they can look very similar. This can make Paget's disease difficult to diagnose. Breast Cancer Care has more on www.breastcancercare.org.uk/upload/pdf/pagets

palliative treatment The use of medical remedies to relieve pain, symptoms, and/or prevent further complications rather than to cure.

pathology The study of disease by the examination of tissues and body fluids under the microscope. A doctor who specializes in pathology is called a pathologist.

photosensitivity Extreme sensitivity to the sun, leaving the patient prone to sunburns. This can be a side effect of some cancer drugs and radiation.

placebo An inert substance, such as a sugar pill. A placebo may be used in clinical trials to compare the effects of a given treatment against no treatment.

platelet One of the three kinds of circulating blood cells. The normal platelet count is about 150,000 to 300,000. Platelets are responsible for creating the first part of the blood clot.

platelet count The number of platelets in a blood sample.

port *Implanted* A catheter connected to a quarter-sized disc that is surgically placed just below the skin in the chest or abdomen. The tube is inserted into a large vein or artery directly into the bloodstream. Fluids, drugs, or blood products can be infused, and blood can be drawn through a needle that is stuck into the disc. Examples: Port-o-cath, Infusaport, Lifeport. *Peritoneal* A catheter connected to a quarter-sized disc that is surgically placed in the abdomen. The catheter is inserted to deliver chemotherapy to the peritoneum (abdominal cavity).

primary tumour The place where a cancer first starts to grow. Even if it spreads elsewhere, it is still known by the place of origin.

progesterone One of the female hormones produced by the ovaries.

progesterone-receptor assay A test that determines if breast cancer is stimulated by the hormone progesterone.

prognosis A statement about the likely outcome of disease in a particular patient. In cancer, it is based on all available information about the type of tumour, staging, therapeutic possibilities, expected results and other personal or medical factors.

prosthesis Artificial replacement of a missing body part.

protocol A treatment plan.

R

radiation therapy X-ray treatment that damages or kills cancer cells.

radical mastectomy Removal of the entire breast along with underlying muscle and the lymph nodes of the armpit (axilla). In a modified radical mastectomy, the underlying (pectoral) muscles are left in place.

radiographer A trained medical specialist, responsible for managing the scanning equipment and obtaining results that are of sufficient quality for the radiologist to make a diagnosis. The radiographer is also responsible for positioning the patient in the correct manner for the best imaging results.

radiologist A doctor with special training in diagnosing diseases by interpreting X-rays and other types of imaging studies. The radiologist will advise the oncologist based on what he or she can determine from the scanning procedures.

recurrence The reappearance of a disease after treatment had caused it to apparently disappear.

recurrent breast cancer Recurrent cancer is cancer that comes back after treatment. Inflammatory breast cancer may come back in the breast (called a local recurrence), in the chest wall, or in another part of the body (called a distant metastasis), including distant organs (such as the lungs or liver), bones, or other lymph nodes.

red blood cells (RBC) Cells in the blood that bring oxygen to tissues and take carbon dioxide from them.

regression The shrinkage of a cancer usually as the result of therapy.

relapse The reappearance of cancer after a disease-free period.

remission The partial or complete shrinkage of cancer usually occurring as the result of therapy. Also a period when the disease is under control. A remission is not necessarily a cure.

risk factor Anything that increases a person's chances of developing cancer, for example, smoking and lung cancer.

S

sarcoma A form of cancer that arises in the supportive tissues, such as bone, cartilage, fat or muscle.

side effects Secondary effects of drugs used for disease treatment.

staging Staging is an agreed and defined classification of the spread of the disease, determined around the time of the initial diagnosis. *Stage I disease* usually indicates that the tumour is confined to the organ of origin when surgical removal of the tumour or organ is likely to be associated with a good prognosis. *Stage IV disease* usually indicates that the tumour has spread widely and the prognosis is less favourable.

stem cells These are primitive cells in marrow that are important in making red and white blood cells and platelets. Generally, the stem cells are largely found in the marrow, but some leave the marrow and circulate in the blood.

steroids A type of hormone.

stomatitis Inflammation and soreness of the mouth. This is sometimes a side effect of chemotherapy or radiation.

surgeon In cancer treatment, the surgeon will be responsible for the removal of the tumour where possible, or to relieve symptoms should the tumour not be removed in its entirety.

systemic Affecting the entire body

systemic disease A disease that affects the entire body not one specific organ.

T

Tamoxifen One of the most widely used hormonal drugs. This drug blocks the effects of oestrogen on many organs, such as the breast. Blocking oestrogen is desirable in some cases of breast cancer because oestrogen promotes their growth. Recent research suggests that tamoxifen may lower the risk of developing breast cancer in women with certain risk factors.

taste alteration A temporary change in taste perception.

theatre The room where your operation takes place.

toxicity Refers to the undesirable and harmful side effects of a drug. Based on the toxicity of a drug, a safe dosage can be determined.

tumour A lump, mass or swelling. A tumour can be benign or malignant.

tumour marker A chemical substance found in increased amounts in the body fluids of some cancer patients. The presence of a tumour marker in the blood for a specific cancer can be an indication that cancer is present in the body. Tumour markers can be used as part of the diagnosis process but generally cannot provide a definitive diagnosis. Tumour markers are also used to monitor the progress of treatment, as well as possible recurrence of cancer after treatment.

U

ultrasound examination The use of high frequency sound waves to aid in diagnosis.

undifferentiated A tumour that appears 'wild' under the microscope, not resembling the tissue of origin. These tumours tend to grow and spread faster than well-differentiated tumours, which do resemble the normal tissue they come from.

urticaria (hives) An allergic reaction marked by itching welts. This may be a side effect of chemotherapy. They may appear at the site of a chemotherapy injection or on other parts of the body.

V

venipuncture Puncturing a vein in order to obtain blood samples, to start an intravenous drip, or to give medication.

vesicant A medication or agent that may cause blistering.

vesicant drugs Chemotherapeutic agents that can cause significant tissue irritation and soreness if they leak outside the vein after injection.

virus A tiny infectious agent that is smaller than bacteria. The common cold is caused by a virus, and the herpes simplex virus causes cold sores.

W

white blood cells (WBC) General term for a variety of cells responsible for fighting invading germs, infection, and allergy-causing agents. Specific white blood cells include granulocytes and lymphocytes.

white blood cell count (WBC count) The actual number of white blood cells seen in a blood sample.

X

X-ray High-energy electromagnetic radiation used to visualize internal body organs to diagnose and treat disease. *See* **radiation therapy.**

Index

skin problems 10, 36, 64, 65, 66, 70, 71, 73-75, 76, 79, 107-111
skincare 75, 81, 136–144, 146
Sloane-Kettering 25
St George's Hospital 21
staging 41, **161**
sun protection 75, 146
support centres 123, 130, 133-4
support groups 122-4, 127, 134, 140
surgery 11, 29, 40–47, 53, 58, 120, 121
symptoms 7, 8, 13-19, 120, 121, 128

T
tamoxifen 63, 64, 67, 68, 71, 75, 88, 120, 121, 135, 143, **162**
taxi cards 117
Taxotere® 37
TeGenero 34
tests (for IBC) 14, 16, 18, 19, 21
The Tech Guys 91
tiredness *see* fatigue
travelling
   help with costs 35, 58
   holidays 38, 103-10, 129
   insurance 105, 106
treatment at home 35
treatment path 22, 28-29
Trick or Treatment 88, 89, 131

U
Udderly Smooth 73, 139, 140

ultrasound 13, 18, **163**
US Food & Drug Administration 86

V
vision *see* eyesight problems
vitamins 67, 73, 85, 99
Vodder massage 53, 80, 121

W
weight gain 36, 72, 76, 99, 120, 121
websites 127-131
Weleda 73, 140
wigs 37, 142
work 70, 121
wound, taking care of 50

X
Xeloda 38